# I Want to Have My Cake & Lose Weight Too

# I Want to Have My Cake & Lose Weight Too

*The Real-Life, Balanced Approach to Managing Your Weight*

Gretchen Lee

ISBN 978-1-257-91207-0

*Dedication*


*For my Mom, Judy Thompson Bauman –*
*Thank you for your inspiring example of*
*unwavering faith and strength,*
*your invaluable wisdom and encouragement*
*and for believing in me.*
*I am most blessed among all daughters.*


*Special thanks to my wonderful family,*
*my Dad, Dr. Harvey Bauman,*
*my sons, Anthony and Nick*
*and countless friends.*

# Contents

# It All Comes Down to Choices

The choice, honestly, is yours. It *is* possible to enjoy some cake and lose weight too. The key lies in *your* personal journey to find balance. After working in multiple wellness settings, I have had the joy to witness hundreds of individuals on their own journeys choose to find balance, practice moderation and adopt a realistic lifestyle approach to weight management.

There is no cookie-cutter solution to managing your weight. Dieting certainly does not work. Each individual must learn to manage their own health risks and special life circumstances with flexibility and patience. So it is up to you, and only you, to decide that you are valuable enough to make some changes.

There is a pretty good chance this isn't the first how-to, weight management, self-help book you've purchased, especially if your weight has contributed to some problems in your life.

Maybe you are the Mom who wonders when she lost herself, her energy and her figure as she's sacrificed herself for her family; the college student who sits alone at the computer, eating because the junk food is simply there; the retired worker, sitting in his favorite chair, watching endless hours of TV out of sheer habit or the exhausted Dad who works two stressful jobs to support his family, with no time to even consider exercise. Where is the balance?

If you have ever found yourself in front of a mirror saying, "How have I let this happen and how do I make this right?" this read is for you.

I have been there too. I know that taking the first, honest step is the hardest part. In addition to the previous questions, these were the most personal to me: Am I going to continue this imbalance – continue to grow larger? Am I going to make choices that will increase my chances of developing the genetic, obesity-related health problems my family history is almost certain to deliver? Will I have to give up the credibility in the career I am so passionate about? Is this the example I want to set for my children?

For me, I *knew* how to be healthy and lose weight. I held a degree in the field, earned additional certifications, took continuing education courses, helped develop wellness programs for physicians and fitness centers and helped guide hundreds of others toward a healthier lifestyle.

Yet, with all that knowledge I continued to gain weight. I finally reached a point of readiness – ready to be honest and value myself enough to get to the bottom of the real issues. Why had I created an unhealthy relationship with food? How had I adopted so many unbalanced habits over time which had led to obesity, medical issues, stress and shame?

My prayer is that you are also *ready* to take an honest and realistic look at your health and are ready to make a change. No one else is going to do it for you. I won't sugar-coat it – change is hard and takes time. Change entails a transformation of your thinking. It involves getting to some core issues of imbalance. It involves an honest evaluation of three distinct areas of self-discovery:

1. What you are saying to yourself
2. The purposeful choices you are making
3. The power you have given away

It is not easy to admit we have been lying to ourselves, but that is exactly what most of us have done and continue to do. We put it off, waiting for the right time while trying to deny and ignore the warning signs.

I, like many of you, needed to find a balance that would accommodate *real life*. I needed to be honest and make real progress that didn't require comparing me to anyone else. What things are in my control and what things are out of my control? Writing this book has allowed me to examine myself, my habits and my excuses. I offer you suggestions that I know work because I practice them myself in my daily, changing life.

I invite you to travel with me through your personal journey of self-discovery that will uncover how certain unbalanced and self-defeating behaviors have become a habitual part of your life. It's time for new, realistic, moderate health-changing habits which will deliver true results.

This book will help you move forward as you:

- Take an honest and realistic look at your health and your priorities
- Let go of all your old diet baggage
- Identify excuses, self-sabotage and barriers that have held you back from facing your own truth
- Educate yourself about your individual, healthier weight range
- Discover the life-changing affects of even a small amount of daily, consistent exercise
- Understand the importance of fueling your body

My biggest hope is that you will learn to accept who you are and your body and become your own best advocate. Get ready to let go of the past that has weighed you down emotionally, physically and spiritually.

As you read, please take note of the * symbol throughout the book. This is a reminder to *write down* what you may be processing from your past and your new goals and behaviors as you move forward.

So, what do you think – can you have a little cake, find the balance to lose weight and keep it off, improve your health and move on with your life too? You can. The choice is yours.

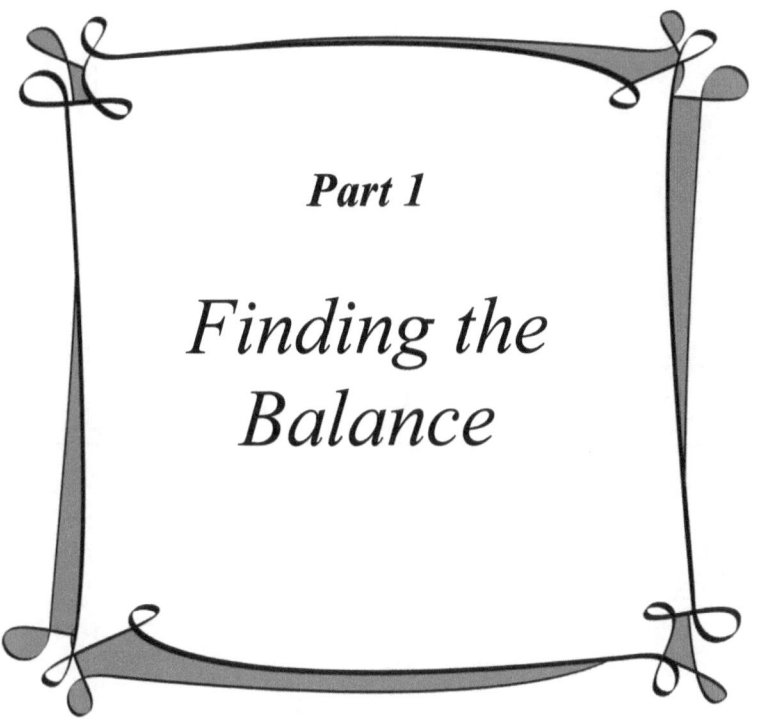

*Part 1*

# *Finding the Balance*

# Chapter 1

# Mind, Body and Spirit

*"You don't have a soul. You are a Soul. You have a body."*
*~ C.S. Lewis*

You are awesome – a unique and miraculous creation. You have been blessed with a body. While you may not be thrilled with some of your insides or outsides, it is the only one you've got for this lifetime. Along with your somewhat genetically predetermined body you have a mind prepped to learn something new every day and a soul with an amazing capacity to give and receive.

Trying to maintain physical, emotional and spiritual balance may seem like an impossible task in today's world. How do you make time for yourself and your health when so many other responsibilities and commitments seem more important? Everyone wants a good quality of life. Sustaining and improving your health in all three areas should be one of your main priorities.

Wellness is described as a journey, not a destination. Your thoughts, beliefs and health choices pave the way for this journey.

Wellness is grounded in the intertwining of the mind, body and spirit and can lend itself to an incredibly broad discussion. For our focus, balanced weight loss and management, we begin with *honesty*.

An honest examination of your mind, body and spirit connection will reveal how it has affected your past weight loss efforts, as well as a renewed awareness of their connection as you develop your own plan for the future. Honesty will serve as your most valuable tool. If you have struggled with your weight and feel you have failed miserably to gain control over this area of your life, take the time to examine all three areas of what makes you, you.

## Mind

Don't you *hate* doing what you know you shouldn't do? Why do we make choices we know are not healthy and why don't we do the things we know will lead to better health? Your choices can be influenced by many factors. We are surrounded by cheap, highly processed and easily accessible "foods." Energy-saving devices reduce our basic daily activities. Sedentary jobs are the norm. Most of us know what we should be doing to live a healthier life, but for one reason or hundreds of excuses, we simply don't. It is a choice.

Rarely have I worked with someone who does not know the basics of what they *should* and *should not* be doing in order to improve their health and lower their weight. I am often thoroughly impressed with the knowledge my clients have in the areas of nutrition and exercise. Wouldn't it be convenient if that knowledge alone could help us sustain a healthy weight? But that is not the case. Believe me, I've tried it.

So, why don't we make better choices when we know better? As with all areas of growth, the journey to understand why you *have not*, *are not* or *do not* choose to make your health a priority is specific to you. I would like to be able to tell you that if you focus all your mental energy and time on weight management you will succeed, but I can't. Real life does not afford us the luxury to make weight loss our only priority.

Your choices are affected by training and experiences from your childhood. They are affected by those you surround yourself with – family, friends, social circles and coworkers. They are affected by your emotions and by your priorities. You are ultimately in control of your priorities, but priorities must change and adapt as your life changes.

To help, begin by *writing down* how you would ultimately like your life priorities to look in the spaces below or in your journal or notebook. Take your time.

What I Would Like My Balanced Priorities to Be:

1. _____
2. _____
3. _____
4. _____
5. _____

Follow this with an honest list of where your priorities realistically lie right now. Are you bound by a work schedule that allows no quality time for family? Are you wasting hours of your day in front of the TV or computer? Tell the truth about how and where you devote yourself, your time and your energy.

My Current Priorities:

1. _____
2. _____
3. _____
4. _____
5. _____

How do your two lists compare? In our minds we know we could be making better choices to improve our quality of life. Learning, and it is a learning process, to prioritize what is truly important and worthwhile to you will lead to a more satisfying life and a better understanding of the control you have and the control you have given away.

I hope that you included your health as one of your top priorities. After all, if you don't have your health, what have you got?

## Body

Myriads of well-intentioned individuals have attempted to lose weight by focusing solely on the body, leaving the mind and spirit out of the equation. I personally feel this issue is why the diet, weight loss and exercise equipment industry draws multiple billions of dollars per year. What scares me the most about this? Some people tend to give away their power and allow someone else to tell them what their physical bodies "need" instead of assuming that control for themselves. After all, that stranger doesn't know you as well as you do. Don't give up your control.

How many of us have allowed ourselves to be convinced that we *need* to join the "elite" gym, we *need* to purchase a particular type of prepackaged food, we *need* to supplement with protein to increase muscle, we *need* to put some pills or shakes in our bodies, we *need* to try this celebrity-endorsed cleanse, or we *need* to purchase that special piece of exercise equipment?

Honestly, our bodies do not *need* any of those things; however we still waste our money and relinquish our power to those who are concerned with our money, not our health.

The infomercials are so convincing. The claims in the muscle magazine sound legitimate. The part-time, pimple-faced employee at the supplement store in the mall claims to have benefitted personally from that $39.95 powdered drink. That piece of exercise equipment has helped hundreds trim inches off of their (you fill in the blank).

The true test comes when the piece of equipment you invested in arrives at your door. Are you actually going to use it? Just because you have money deducted from your checking account to pay your gym membership every month doesn't get you to the gym. What happens when you stop eating the prepackaged meals and return to your old eating habits? How about the slap in the face when you realize your fluorescent yellow urine is actually that $39.95 supplement being flushed down the toilet?

If your goal is a healthy body, recognize your mental and spiritual connection to it. The saying, "My heart just wasn't in it," has nothing to do with your physical anatomy. It signals a disconnect between the mind, body and spirit. Focusing your energy on pushing your body without this vital connection will only prove to serve as a temporary fix to a much broader issue. I will share much more information about what your body does need to function optimally later.

## Spirit

Do you feel lost and out of control? Does your current state make you feel stressed or depressed? Some may place these emotions under the area of the mind, but I feel they reach much deeper. It is time to recognize the connection between your spirit and your health.

When your soul feels empty you will not be the best person you can be. It is even more difficult to take care of and serve those around you when you are spiritually empty. We, as humans, need to acknowledge something larger than ourselves and the necessity to fill our spiritual tanks daily.

The most common reply we hear today in response to, "How are you doing?" is, "Busy." I am often guilty of this myself. We have allowed ourselves to become so busy that we not only neglect to make time to properly care for ourselves and allow our spirit to be filled, but have given much of our power away. I would like to stress that you have more control over your health than you think you do.

I propose that the growing waistlines of our nation and others, who have adopted our sedentary lifestyle and unhealthy eating habits, are much more of a spirit and soul issue than anything else.

## How to Fill Your Spiritual Tank

*"Balance, peace, and joy are the fruit of a successful life.*
*It starts with recognizing your talents and finding*
*ways to serve others by using them."*
*~ Thomas Kinkade*

Use these points to maintain a balanced spirit:

- Recognize the connection your spirit has to your mind and body.
  When you balance these three areas in your life, reevaluate your priorities and take back the control you have given away to make the time to improve your health daily, the benefits will *astound* you. You simply feel better; depression, stress and anxiety diminish. You stop comparing yourself to others and recognize your value as an individual – no matter what size or shape you are.

- Pray and meditate
  Set aside time each day to be quiet and breathe. Thank God for your blessings, ask for guidance and believe that your prayers will be answered.

- Take care of yourself
  Believe me, I know personally that this is much easier said than done. You will be a much better parent, employee, spouse and friend when you take care of your own basic needs. One of the best ways to do this is to make daily exercise a necessary part of most of your days. Even a few minutes a day will *change* your life.

- Ask for help
  When you genuinely need it, ask for help from your family, friends, church or a local community support system. Accept the help with appreciation and do not feel guilty about it.

- Serve someone else
  Look for an area or place where your gifts can fill someone else's spirit. You can choose to sit back and watch life pass you by or get up and get involved to make a difference in the world around you. Using your gifts to serve others will fill your soul.

- Show gratitude
  Let those around you know how much they mean to you. Do not let the opportunity pass. Seize it, whenever it arises, to tell and show someone that you appreciate them.

- Forgive
  Give forgiveness not only for the person or circumstance that has caused you pain, but forgive for yourself. Let it go. The peace gained by forgiving will free you to move forward.

## Recognizing Balance and Imbalance

Do you recognize imbalance when you see it? Many of us, albeit painful to admit, prefer to remain in a state of denial about our weight and our health. We want what we want and keep our heads in the sand about all the rest.

For example, have you ever eaten a whole bag of some food item, like chips or candy? You knew at one level that eating the whole bag was unbalanced, but did that stop you from eating it? The fact that you purchased the bag in the first place, knowing full well you would most likely eat the whole thing, would be the better place to begin.

Far too many of us believe the ads we see in stores and on television, the radio, in magazines and on the internet. We *want* to believe it! We all know that, "If it sounds too good to be true, it probably is." But when it comes to losing weight we ignore common sense, pick up the phone, grab the credit card and dial that toll free number in hopes of "losing those inches fast!"

Have you ever taken a close look at the microscopic print at the bottom of the TV screen under those airbrushed photos? If you haven't, I'll paraphrase what 99% of them state: *Results not typical. Participants also followed a reduced calorie and exercise program.* Even though you have to grab a magnifying glass to see it, at least the truth is stated somewhere among all the hype. If this same phrase is stated in practically all of the ads and infomercials, doesn't it make sense that *eating smarter* and *moving more* are probably the keys to managing your weight?

I am consistently impressed at how advertisers use paid actors or public personalities to promote their wares. A balanced view will recognize that a television personality may not be the best expert in the exercise field. That person gets paid to endorse a product that may or may not be responsible for their great-looking body. Using that piece of equipment does not mean you will use it when it arrives at your home or that you will ever achieve a size 4 figure. When stated clearly we see that our balanced reasoning sometimes escapes us.

Learning to look for and identify the balance in any given situation is integral to moving forward. Our American lifestyle doesn't leave a lot of room for balance. We do not want to have to work hard for something as important as our health because we're working so hard in every other part of our lives.

The mind, body and spirit connection cannot be minimized on your journey to improve your health. As you notice imbalance in one or all of these areas, *write it down.* Consider the steps you can take to balance the scales a little more and then take action. Make the time to learn what small changes will work in your life and you will see the benefits which will lead your healthy spirit to a healthy mind and body.

## To Sum Up

My hope is that you will take a closer look at your daily life and begin to determine some small ways to find more balance. *No one* is perfect and *no one* will ever get it completely right, but striving for balance a little every day will make all the difference in your mind, body and spirit.

# Chapter 2

# Honesty and Readiness

*"The greatest gift you ever give is your honest self."*
*~ Mr. Fred Rogers*

Let's be honest. The first step in making any real, personal change is to take responsibility for where you are right here, right now.

At this moment, can you honestly say you are satisfied with the state of your body and your health? Has being overweight led to various health problems? Are you no longer able to fit into some or most of your clothes? Are you waiting to lose the weight so you can buy new clothes? Do you lack the energy to do the things you would like to do?

It is often painful to take a realistic look at where we find ourselves. Maybe you're saying, "How did I get here? How could I have let this happen?" or, "Do I still have toes down there?!" Taking an honest look in this very moment is the *only* place to start.

Years ago a dear, elderly friend challenged me on this point. She told me, "If you tell someone your job is to help people lose weight, they are never going to believe you." She delivered some hard-to-hear, tough love. I was 36 years old, 5' 2", squeezing (I mean really squeezing) into a size 14 and 185+ pounds (I stopped weighing myself after I reached 185). You would not have picked me out of a line-up as the weight-loss professional.

I had focused my education and career around helping others in the one area of my life in which I privately struggled – weight management. I worked at trying to keep the extra weight off, even succeeding for a few years at a time, only to lose my balance as different life stages and trials arose. No one was making my choices for me. I was perpetuating habits and behaviors that hurt my mind, body and spirit. Those choices had to change in order for me to move forward. My prayer is that you will also take the time to have a heart-to-heart with yourself. It is time to be honest.

## See it in Writing

You've heard me stress the importance of keeping a journal along your journey. Now is the time. Get out that pen and paper and start writing!

- Record what you are eating and drinking.
- Record how much planned exercise you are getting in, even if only 5 or 10 minutes.
- Record moments of success and moments where you get off track from a healthier lifestyle.
- Examine your habits and record what you are beginning to uncover about your choices.

It is difficult to lie to yourself when you see the details of your choices recorded in your own hand. It may seem time-consuming to follow up after yourself and keep track of the details, but I encourage you to give it a try, even if only for one week. It is a powerful tool in your journey to develop lasting change.

Find a way to track your choices that works for you and your lifestyle. If you know writing in a notebook or journal isn't something you will be consistent at, try an alternative approach:

- An online site like www.sparkpeople.com. This valuable site helps you set up your individualized plan, record your choices and receive balanced advice.
- Text yourself.
- Set up a private blog for your eyes only.
- Set up a public blog, share it with your friends and ask them for their support along your journey.
- Tweet yourself throughout your day, review your thread and look for patterns.

Choose one of these forms of record-keeping that appeals to you and go for it! I promise this will be one of the most enlightening efforts you can do for yourself.

## Reality

*"We either create our own reality
or allow someone else to do it for us."*
~ J.J. Dewey

Developing a healthier and more balanced lifestyle requires a firm grounding in reality. If you are like every other person who has ever attempted to lose a fair amount of weight, you are holding on to strong opinions, misinformation and false ideas regarding weight loss. It is practically impossible to go through the day without being bombarded with unfounded and untrue information from TV ads, infomercials, books, magazines and diet plans. Many people have difficulty separating truth from fiction.

Reality is based in facts. It brings with it a heaping dose of honesty and accountability that is often hard to face. Many of us do not want to accept that losing weight and improving our quality of life takes time and effort. We do not want to give up the search for the *fast*, *simple* and *easy* diet. Cheap, high-calorie, high-fat and easily accessible convenience foods don't make it any easier when trying to change to a healthier lifestyle.

I'll tell it to you straight: there is no *secret* to losing weight and keeping it off. There is no *simple* or *fast* solution. There is no *magic pill* or *easy* workout program. If there were, we would all be popping it or doing it. Weight loss seems, for many, overwhelmingly difficult so it is understandable that many look for the easy route.

Remember that it takes effort to maintain a healthy weight. It takes time management, commitment and a sincere desire to improve your quality of life. All of these components must be coupled with a realistic plan to handle what life offers up each day.

The term, "take care of yourself" may seem like an exclusive luxury for the wealthy when your time and energy are focused on daily survival. Nonetheless, it is possible and worth every bit of effort. *You* are worth the effort. Discovering what will work for you will help you deal with and enhance everything else you have on your plate. Remind yourself of this reality during your journey and resolve to seek the truth.

## Being Overweight is *Okay*?

How have we come to accept being overweight as the norm? Why do we tell ourselves it is okay? We know intellectually it is unhealthy to be overweight, yet the trend of expanding waistlines continues. A recent study also confirmed that our perception is changing regarding what is considered heavy. As more and more people carry extra, unhealthy pounds they are more likely to view their weight as normal and don't feel the need to lose weight. (1)

The big question – How do we change this perception when two-thirds of adults and one-third of our nation's children are overweight? Here in the South there are many who seem to have accepted that being overweight, with the accompanying health problems, is an expected part of life. People talk about their "sugar" (Type 2 Diabetes), and discuss all the medications they are on for their heart conditions and their upcoming doctor's appointments all while smoking a cigarette and drinking a large soda.

Many have given their power and responsibility away by becoming dependent on conventional medicine. "Hey, it doesn't matter what I do to my body, there is a pill for that."

Choices, people, choices! No wonder we see our next generation of children growing larger even faster than the last and developing diseases we used to see only in adults.

How many "reality" shows focus on weight loss and dieting? If we choose to tune in we see participants struggling mentally and physically to take off hundreds of pounds. The personal trainers scream, the weight melts off at 15 or more pounds each week. Who will succeed? Who will fail? Who will be voted off? Our overweight culture has now become popular evening entertainment.

Recently these same shows have started to address the fact that some of the participants gain the majority if not all the weight back when they return to their *real* homes, families and jobs. This correlates exactly with what we see in the weight management field. It's just like dieting – a few will commit to some form of lifestyle change, while most revert back to their old inactive lifestyles, eating behaviors and habits because the initial weight loss was not under real-life conditions. And while I am glad many of the participants in these programs learn to eat healthier and exercise, the settings and circumstances are *far from reality*.

The more accurate reality show might play out like this: A 40-year-old single Mom pushes the button of her alarm clock before the crack of dawn, works out to her exercise video, rushes to shower and dress, wakes up her kids for school, makes breakfast and lunches, drops the kids off at school, drives to work, *writes down* what she eats throughout her day in the little tablet she keeps tucked in her purse and aims for a pound of weight loss in the week.

This Mom then picks up her kids, takes them with her to help with the grocery shopping where she helps them distinguish between choosing affordable yet nourishing foods and tries to make time in the evening to play outside with them in between all of the homework, sports, household chores and responsibilities. Then the next day starts all over again. This scenario hardly makes for exciting and entertaining television, does it? But *that* is reality.

Examine your mindset about this and raise your standards for your health. You are worth it.

## Examine Your Readiness to Change

"It just clicked."
"It was time."
"I made up my mind that something had to change."

These are honest statements I have heard from individuals who made the choice to adopt a balanced lifestyle to manage their weight. It is remarkable to see the mind-shift in someone who is truly ready to adopt a healthier lifestyle. Does this mean they gave up desserts for life and became skinny people? Far from it; oftentimes the biggest change was balancing their thinking about what their realistic, healthy lifestyle would entail. That then led to their understanding of what a healthy weight range would realistically mean for them. On that foundation they then made small changes that, in time, led to big results.

Some people hit rock bottom when their health issues force them to become ready. Others simply decide they are tired of listening to their own excuses. Many parents and grandparents reach this point when they are unable to enjoy simple activities with their kids and grandchildren.

Where are you in your readiness to change? Ask yourself, "Am I honestly ready to move forward and commit to making balanced changes in order to improve my health?" Let's face it, life will never offer the perfect or ideal time to start a journey to your healthier weight range, but recognizing what stands in your way and clearing as many obstacles as possible will create a much smoother path ahead.

Please thoughtfully read over and answer each of the questions in the following *Readiness Questionnaire* to explore how ready you are to make some significant changes in your daily life. It will be helpful to *write down* the honest thoughts that come into your mind after reading each question.

## Readiness Questionnaire

1. Am I motivated to make *long-term*, lifestyle changes?
2. Am I ready to begin making healthier eating choices and choosing appropriate portion sizes of foods?
3. Am I really ready to make a *permanent* change?
4. Am I willing to look back and honestly examine past successes and failures?
5. Am I committed to discovering what type of exercise(s) fit my lifestyle and set aside time *almost every day* for exercise?
6. Am I ready to give up dieting and the pursuit of the quick-fix in exchange for more balanced, manageable, daily habits?
7. Do I believe that a slower approach to weight loss is the better choice?

8.  Do I love and respect myself enough to keep going during times of trial and return as quickly as I can to the healthy lifestyle habits I have worked to develop if I fall behind?
9.  Am I actively working through, with help and support, my unresolved issues relating to food addiction, excessive emotional eating or past issues contributing to my weight problem?
10. Are there distractions or significant changes in my life that may challenge my commitment to a healthier lifestyle?
11. Are my weight loss goals realistic?

If you answered a resounding, "YES!" to these questions, then you are at a healthier starting point for your journey.

Answering "No" to even one of these should give you a moment of pause. What can you do to change that response? Is it out of your control? You may be able to change some factors, but possibly not others.

Every one of us can commit to small, manageable behavior changes. As we continue to sift our thoughts and choices through the sieve of reality, it helps to remember that there will never be a perfect time to begin. Each of us has a long list of obstacles, unique to our own lives that could stand in our way.

Readiness – that thing that just "clicks" – can mean the difference between the positive experience of developing new, healthier habits versus trying to force something which simply will not and cannot succeed. Some of the factors preventing readiness may be outside of your realm of control. Again, identify what things you have in your power to change.

If you answered "no" to a few of the questions there are ways to increase your readiness. Start by seeing your doctor. I recommend all of my clients complete a full physical, including blood work, as they begin to adopt a healthier lifestyle. Use this to educate yourself about what is going on with your body right now. You can use this as a baseline for a comparison as you establish daily, healthier habits over time. If you haven't had a physical in a few years you may be surprised at how your readiness may change after uncovering risk factors you have been trying to ignore.

## Identifying Food Addiction and Emotional Eating

In the pursuit to move forward in honesty, consider a serious issue which may be hindering your progress. One of the readiness questions above deals with addiction or imbalance in one's relationship with food. The topic of food addiction stirs some debate. Some question whether developing an addiction to something essential to survival is even possible. It is possible.

People who suffer from a food addiction experience many of the same physical and psychological triggers as other addicts. But unlike those struggling with alcohol and drug addictions, who must completely eliminate those substances from their lives as part of their recovery, the food addict cannot eliminate and avoid food as part of his or her healing. The food addict has to choose balance while having to contend with food repeatedly during each and every day of their lives.

Consider carefully your relationship with food. Do you reach for food as a way to cope with life issues, even as someone else might reach for cigarettes, alcohol or drugs? Putting food in your mouth to fill a void in your life simply does not work. The comfort is very short-lived because even though you may *feel* comforted for a moment, you are not actually comforted. It is simply a feeling.

You must learn to differentiate between the feeling and realistically solving the issue. And because these short-term fixes are not realistically fixing anything there is shame afterwards. Just like an alcoholic might regret their indulgence during a hangover, someone with an unbalanced relationship with food always regrets the binge later. Guilt, regret and shame are common words associated with food addiction.

Dr. Ramani Durvasula, PhD, a practicing psychologist in California, personally battled food addiction for years and recently shared her personal struggle. She offers the following summary to assist as you take an honest look at your relationship with food.

### Warning Signs of Food Addiction

1. You hide food in your car, home or office.
2. You think about food more than 1 hour per day.

3. You eat after arguing with a spouse or friend.
4. You experience withdrawal symptoms when you're not eating.
5. You cannot stop eating, even when you're not hungry.

Again, the one feeling associated with this unbalanced relationship with food – shame. Trying to deal with emotional upheavals or difficult life circumstances with food is just as futile as dealing with problems with drugs and alcohol. Dr. Durvasula offers the following advice for those who can identify.

- Solution #1: Understand that food will *not* solve any of the following emotions…
  F – Frustration
  L – Loneliness
  A – Anxiousness
  B – Boredom

- Solution #2: Keep a daily food log and *write down* not only what, when and where you are eating, but the feelings associated with it.

- Solution #3: Review your food journal to identify emotional or stress-induced eating. This will help you identify eating and binging triggers and help you become more self-aware.

One of the best choices you can make when dealing with emotional eating is to reach out to a friend or support group. I say this as a former lonely eater. When depressed and lonely I reached for food to fill that void. Initially it would make me feel good, but I felt ashamed and disappointed with myself afterwards. There is the common denominator again – shame.

I finally realized this habit had been sabotaging my weight loss attempts for over two decades. Only then did I reach out for support; specifically from my sister, Stephanie, who also struggled with maintaining a healthy weight. Even though we live on opposite coasts, we encourage each other by phone. Now, instead of sitting in front of the TV snacking at night after my kids go to bed, I call Stephanie.

It is time to ask yourself, "Do I use food to try to fill a void or deal with stress?" If you can identify with a food addiction problem, or are an emotional eater, I encourage you to reach out for help. You need someone on your side who can provide non-judgmental guidance, encouragement and support. Find a relative or friend with whom you can be brutally honest and ask them for help.

You may find the services of a mental health professional or support group incredibly helpful. There are local chapters of Overeaters Anonymous in almost every city. Realize you are not alone and take action to adopt a healthier perspective about food and eating.

## To Sum Up

If you want to succeed in managing your weight, begin your personal journey based in reality – your life's honest reality. Make the effort to educate yourself to find out what works for you personally. Truthfully examine your relationship with food. Understand that food will not and cannot help you deal with emotional highs and lows.

As you focus on lifestyle change, prepare to ride the ebb and flow of what your life may deliver. Be honest with yourself and prepare for a good dose of eye-opening reality. You can do it!

# Chapter 3

# Why Diets Don't Work

*"The second day of a diet is always easier than the first.*
*By the second day you're off of it."*
~ Jackie Gleason

I love Weight Watchers' ad campaign, "Diets Don't Work – *Weight Watchers* Does." The first time I saw the commercial slogan I ran to the TV and shouted, "Yes!" at the screen. Why was I so excited? Because diets *don't* work! This nugget of wisdom is exactly what we in the wellness field have been preaching for decades. Countless studies and thousands of individual testimonials back this up.

I commend Weight Watchers for stating this truth and for providing an affordable and reality based weight management program. Why do support group programs like Weight Watchers help so many reach a healthier weight range and learn to maintain it? They focus on permanent lifestyle change through the development of small, healthier, manageable, real-life daily habits.

The truth is, however, that even though many people find success through such programs, some still gain their weight back after spending time and money on them. When I began working in weight management fifteen years ago, I was eager to discover why those individuals who achieved initial success with balanced programs did not stick with it. To my surprise, I found one common issue haunting practically every person who had made a serious attempt to lose weight and maintain it: diet baggage.

## Diet Baggage

The constant push to diet is *everywhere*. Designers of some weight-loss programs cash in on popular demands for the easiest and fastest route to lose weight. Have you glanced at the magazines at the grocery store check-out line lately? Dieting sells. Sadly, many who are on the endless dieting cycle are easy targets to the latest diet gimmick. As long as there are desperate people out there looking for the quick fix, there will be those who are eager to make a buck off of their desperation.

Most diets require unrealistic, unmanageable and temporary behaviors which cannot be maintained over the course of a lifetime. For the most part, diets are extremely restrictive and cannot adapt to our real lives. How many of us can relate to the term, "yo-yo dieting?" It describes the vicious cycle of losing and gaining weight over and over again.

Here is an interesting statistic for you to consider – 80-90% of traditional dieters gain *all the weight back*, often accompanied by fifteen additional pounds or more. You've probably seen or experienced this for yourself. I have not only done it, but have witnessed relatives and friends over the years repeat the process over and over.

If you look back at your previous weight loss attempts you probably have a list of brief successes followed by relapses which inevitably led to feelings of failure and depression. A mental review of your dieting history may reveal that you bypassed the real issues to jump on the "quick-fix" bandwagon. Consider this as I provide you with the following summary.

## Diet Review

- Liquid Shakes
  Reducing your daily calories by drinking a couple of sugar-laden or artificially sweetened shakes may help you lose weight, but what happens after you stop drinking the shakes and return to eating a few meals a day?

Years ago I committed to one of the popular weight loss shake diets. I tried to stick to it, but eventually I grew tired of liquid meals and could not fight the urge to chew on something. I ended up following each shake with a normal, sound meal. Over the course of a few weeks I gained five pounds! There are medically supervised programs which do involve reduced calorie shakes for the severely overweight who need to lose weight in order to literally save their lives, but if they are not accompanied by a balanced, sound lifestyle change program the end result is similar to any other diet program.

- Home delivered, reduced calorie meals
  These have been part of the weight-loss industry for decades, but have recently gained new popularity. Admittedly, this diet plan is very convenient. Entire meals come to your front door. No need to cook, count calories, measure portions or read labels. These positive aspects also have a negative flip side: If your goal is lifetime weight management, can you purchase and eat those meals for the rest of your life?

Just like any other diet plan, users of convenience food diets typically gain the weight back once they stop ordering these meals. The average individual simply cannot afford it.

- Over-the-Counter Diet Pills
  Herbal and over-the-counter weight loss aids have been around for a long time. The industry continues to prosper year after year, promising the fastest and easiest weight loss possible.

The truth is that diet pills are a complete waste of money. Yes, you may lose weight, but unless you change your eating and exercise habits, you will gain the weight back as soon as you stop taking the pills.

Most diet supplements work by tricking the body into thinking it is not hungry. Some contain caffeine and other stimulants that supposedly boost metabolism and increase energy levels.

Aside from their ineffectiveness for long-term weight loss, there are legitimate concerns regarding the safety of diet pills. Reported side effects range from high blood pressure, increased heart rate and heart palpitations to mood alteration, headaches and sleep problems. Do not be fooled! The pills will not help you in the long run.

- Diuretics, Colon Cleansers and Weight-Loss Teas
  Among the "weight loss" aids on store shelves are products that temporarily reduce weight by removing water from the body.

  Again, any results you attain from using diuretics, laxatives or cleansers will not last. The weight you lose will not be fat, regardless of the claims on the packaging. These products only remove water – that is all. Excessive use can cause serious harm by lowering blood pressure and depleting the body of much needed electrolytes.

## The Lone Dieter

I would like to address a specific group of dieters who are honestly trying to make healthier choices. Mom and Dad have you made this statement? "I have decided to lose weight and cook healthier meals, but it is hard to cook two meals for my family." My response is always, "Why would you cook or purchase a healthy meal for yourself and not one for the rest of your household? You don't want them to be healthy too?"

The idea that maybe it would be best for the entire family to change to a healthier way of eating is *completely* foreign to some dieters. They have decided that eating healthier, which to them often means a restrictive, unappealing diet because of their own baggage, is not something they want to put the rest of their family through. Instead of making moderate changes for the whole family the dieter falls into the restrictive deprivation mode while the kids and spouse have their daily desserts, sodas and fried foods.

It is time to develop new habits that will benefit *everyone*. If you hold the role as main food preparer or shopper in your family or household, work on letting go of your old baggage so your whole family can benefit.

## Help! I Don't Know How to Keep the Weight Off!

I completed one of my internships with a group of gifted physicians, nurses, registered dieticians and exercise physiologists in Charlotte, NC. The doctors there conducted studies using a combination of prescribed medications coupled with behavior modification. Although the concept of medication-assisted weight loss is controversial, for many severely overweight individuals, the addition of medications when partnered with a physician-supervised lifestyle change program can be effective. This was my first opportunity to focus on weight management with a professional team approach. I learned so much working alongside those in the medical, nutrition and exercise fields.

After completing this internship and my degree I was at a routine annual visit with my physician. I noticed that the nurse, Cindy, whom I had known for quite a few years, had lost a significant amount of weight. We began chatting about her weight loss and I mentioned the internship I had just completed. Cindy quickly turned and closed the door. She told me that she had been receiving a prescription for the same medications from a local physician, but feared gaining all of the weight back as soon as the prescription ran out. Cindy admitted that she had not changed *any* eating or exercise habits.

She was right to be concerned about gaining back the most significant amount of weight she had ever lost. While writing down the name of the local doctor, she implored me to speak with him about adding a behavior modification aspect to the medication regimen for the patients in his weight loss program.

That week I walked into that doctor's office, sat down and asked him how many of his patients he had to start back on the medications because they had regained all of their weight. Of course the majority of them, he said, had gained the weight back as soon as the prescription ran out. I proposed a lifestyle-focused, nutrition, exercise and behavior modification program for all of his patients currently on the weight-loss medication regimen. He agreed and hired me on the spot.

Patients who were only interested in receiving the medications and a quick-fix, even those who would have benefitted from losing a large amount of weight, were respectfully declined from entering the weight loss program. Individuals who were taking the medications who had never tried to manage their weight through healthier eating and exercise, however, were offered this new supervised lifestyle program.

The vast majority of patients, including Cindy, were *thrilled* to participate. Not only did they receive instruction about eating smarter and developing a consistent exercise program, but they received months of behavior modification coaching as they adopted a balanced, healthier lifestyle. In time, many of the participants voluntarily asked to stop taking the medications.

## Let it Go

If you honestly want to be healthy and manage your weight then *stop dieting*. Let it go. Commit to removing that four-letter word from your vocabulary all together. Dieting will not solve your problems and in fact may undermine your efforts to develop a balanced, life-changing perspective. Your time and energy are too valuable, *you* are too valuable, to head in the wrong direction.

Regardless of the route dieters take, diets only work for the short-term. I hope anyone who still believes in dieting will consider this: What is being thrown in our faces through advertising and marketing is not making us healthier. It is time to stop funding the billion dollar diet bandwagon.

It may be hard to resist each new gimmick to lose weight, especially if you have ridden the diet roller coaster for a while. But you know what you need to do: Now is the time to be honest and stand on your own. You have all that you need to succeed. Trust in that reality.

## To Sum Up

Despite the hundreds, possibly thousands of diets available, you would think obesity rates would stop rising, or at least slow down. They continue to increase every year, especially among our children. Be honest with yourself and realize that a change in small, consistent, healthier habits will deliver realistic, long-term success. Diets don't work.

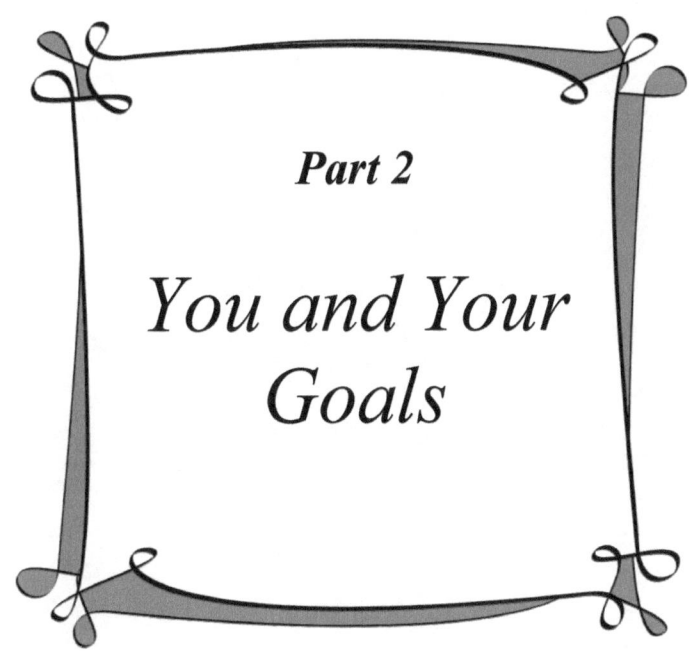

*Part 2*

# You and Your Goals

# Chapter 4

# Acceptance and Wisdom

*"God, grant me the serenity to accept the things I cannot*
*change, the courage to change the things I can,*
*and the wisdom to know the difference."*
*~ Reinhold Niebuhr*

During your journey, I encourage you to recall the above prayer often. Read it slowly aloud a few times and think about its meaning: The root of this prayer acknowledges desire for help and support. We need a revelation from God and awareness beyond our limited view. This prayer has great value for anyone invested in the goal of weight loss and maintenance.

There are "things" and people in your life you will not be able to change nor control. Yet recognize, whether you feel it right now or not, that you do have control over many "things" you can change.

A look in the mirror is usually all it takes to see the person typically responsible for the design, construction and maintenance of the roadblocks in our lives. I have seen it both in my life and in my role as a Wellness Coach. Maybe, during this honest process, you are beginning to discover that YOU are your own biggest barrier. It is hard to admit and take responsibility for this, but that is exactly what you must do in order to move forward. Own it, accept it, then choose to do something about it.

As you read through this chapter focus on the details. Identify each choice you make that contributes to your weight and health issues. Examine your daily habits, healthy and unhealthy. The following section will walk you through these areas and help you determine what is and is not within your control.

## Getting Personal

Use the space below to fill in some personal information. Fill in your name and your current age and weight. Follow by filling in what you weighed at different stages of your life. How much did you weigh on your wedding day? If you have children, record what you weighed before and after each pregnancy. Maybe your weight changed dramatically after going through menopause or after a serious injury, illness or surgery. Record significant life events and your weight before and after.

Full Name _____

Current Age_____          Current Weight_____

Weight as a teenager or at HS graduation_____

Age 20_____          Age 30_____

Age 40_____          Age 50_____

Age 60_____          Age 70_____

Other important stages or changes:

_____
_____
_____
_____
_____

List sports or activities you were involved in during various stages of your life. Maybe you played sports while in school or had a health club membership. Did you have a job that required you to be active and walk? Maybe you were a healthy weight before you started working at the fast food restaurant, chose a sedentary computer career or job that required you to travel and sit for long periods of time. Recognize the role activity or lack of activity played in the various stages of your life.

Now list your past weight loss attempts. Maybe you dieted on your own or joined a group for support. Record the date, beginning weight, ending weight and how long you were able to maintain your weight loss. Give a best guess if you do not remember exactly.

| Month/Year | Self or Assisted Program | Results |
|---|---|---|
|  |  |  |
|  |  |  |
|  |  |  |
|  |  |  |

Now examine what you have recorded.

First, notice your name. In all likelihood it does not read, "Cindy Crawford, Super Model," "Arnold Schwarzenegger, former Mr. Universe" or one of the actors from that vampire movie series the teens are all crazy about. You should not and cannot compare yourself to anyone else. Your name carries with it your personal history and all the past generations on both sides of your family – good and bad. You have your ancestors to thank for many things that make you who you are. Many of them are positive and some are likely negative.

Do you see patterns? Many parents, both Moms and Dads, gain weight after the birth of each child. This is quite common. Not only do our priorities change after having kids, but the time we set aside to care for ourselves decreases substantially.

Once you have completed your weight-loss history, search for what has worked for you and what has not. Look at how changes in your circumstances or family status impacted your weight.

Most importantly, use this information to help you move forward. Don't dwell on the past, but do learn from it.

## Your Health and Family History

Carrying too much extra weight destroys your health over time. Improving your health does not realistically need to be your *only* reason for losing weight, but it should be a priority. Your overall health and quality of life are closely intertwined.

Good quality of life has varying dimensions, but for the most-part it describes your level of independence, self-care and the ability to do the things you want to do. Making consistently unhealthy choices increases your risk for disease and makes it very difficult to maintain good quality of life. This fact should resonate more if you know there is a genetic propensity toward certain diseases in your family.

Wellness Coaching is not a common career so I often get the question, "What is a Wellness Coach and why did you decide to go into that field?" First I explain that the field of wellness is focused not only on prevention of disease and reduction of disease risks, but living a balanced and optimal life through healthier choices. I commonly share that my personal family history of disease was also an encouraging factor. My Dad's side has a history of heart disease. My Mom's side of the family struggled with everything imaginable – heart disease, stroke, cancer, diabetes, Alzheimer's and obesity.

Working with cardiac rehabilitation patients has clarified for me the genetic factors related to heart disease. On my first day working at a cardiac rehabilitation fitness center, I expected to see a room full of overweight individuals. I was shocked, however, to see that almost half of the members were well within a healthy weight range.

Even my own father, a retired business man and professor and one of the fittest men you could ever meet, was diagnosed with heart disease at 72. This was a man who had operated his own mountain landscaping business for many years and meticulously maintained his weight and a healthy diet. Yet he began feeling tightness in his chest and wisely saw his cardiologist. My very active, healthy Dad turned out to need a six-way heart bypass due to several near-total blockages and damage from a past heart attack he had not even noticed!

My Dad's doctors explained that he was dealing with a genetic heart condition. The only reason he had not dropped dead of a massive heart attack was due to his incredible fitness level.

I use this example to help you understand that there are certain genetic factors you have absolutely no control over. It demonstrates why we not only need to have a healthy lifestyle, but need to have yearly physicals and discuss our family history with our physicians.

The fact that my Dad made his health and fitness a priority was one of the factors that saved his life.

Take a moment to record some of your own family history. Call a relative who may give you some insight into your genetically related health issues.

- Do you currently have unhealthy risk factors? (high blood pressure, high cholesterol, diabetes, poor diet, physical inactivity, smoking, etc.)

_____

_____

_____

_____

- Are there serious genetic health concerns in your family history that will increase your risk? (premature heart disease, cancer, diabetes, arthritis, etc.)

Direct Relative                    Health Issue

_____

_____

_____

_____

All genetic risk factors aside, being overweight increases your risk for:

- High Blood Pressure
  Although it is normal for blood pressure to increase with age, if you have a family history of high blood pressure or heart disease, being overweight will most definitely increase your risk. Most people who are only moderately overweight often have high-normal to moderately high blood pressure.

- High LDL (bad) Cholesterol
  Cholesterol is a type of fat that circulates in your bloodstream. Low density lipoprotein (LDL) is the main source of cholesterol build-up and blockage in the arteries of the heart.

- Low HDL (good) Cholesterol
  High density lipoprotein (HDL) helps keep cholesterol from building up in the walls of the arteries of the heart.

- High levels of triglycerides
  Triglycerides are the most common form of fat in the body. A lot of those extra calories you take in are converted to triglycerides and stored as fat.

- Coronary Heart Disease
  CHD is a condition in which a substance called plaque builds up inside the coronary arteries. These arteries supply oxygen-rich blood to your heart. Plaque is made up of fat, cholesterol, calcium, and other substances found in your blood. Plaque can narrow or block the coronary arteries and reduce blood flow to the heart muscle. This can cause angina (chest pain or discomfort) or a heart attack.

- Heart Failure
  This is a serious condition in which the heart cannot pump enough blood to the meet the body's needs.

- Stroke
  The heavier you are the greater your risk of having a stroke, specifically an ischemic stroke. An ischemic stroke occurs when the blood vessels supplying the brain are blocked.

- Osteoarthritis
  This is a slow wearing away of the joints, usually involving the knees, hips and lower back. Being only

10 pounds overweight can increase the force on each knee by 30-60 pounds with each step. (1) Is it any wonder that being overweight is one of the main reasons for primary joint replacement?

- Gallbladder Disease
  Your gallbladder is a small, pear shaped organ that assists your liver in the storage of bile. When the bile hardens it creates gall stones and can lead to gallbladder disease. A diet full of fatty foods and low fiber greatly increases this risk.

- Sleep Apnea and Respiratory problems
  Excess weight can lead to sleep apnea which is a serious condition that causes someone to actually stop breathing for short periods during sleep. This can deprive the heart muscle of oxygen. Excess weight can also cause excessive snoring. Not only is this disruptive to a normal nighttime sleep pattern, but causes sleepiness and lack of energy during the day.

- Some Cancers
  In women these include cancer of the uterus, gallbladder, cervix, ovary, breast and colon. Overweight men are at greater risk of developing cancer of the colon, rectum and prostate.

- Type 2 Diabetes
  The foods you eat are broken down into proteins, fats and carbohydrates. The carbohydrates, that are high in foods like fruit and bread, are broken down further into a sugar called glucose. Glucose goes into your blood to produce energy. Your pancreas produces a hormone called insulin which helps to move the glucose from the blood to the cells. Type 2 diabetes develops when the insulin produced does not work properly and cannot move the glucose into the cells.

The incidence of Type 2 diabetes continues to increase and accounts for 90-95% of all cases. The increase coincides directly with our country's expanding waistlines and physical inactivity. An estimated 21 million people in the U.S. are currently diagnosed with diabetes with another 54 million diagnosed as pre-diabetic, meaning they have elevated, fasting blood sugar levels; borderline Type 2 diabetics. Although Type 2 diabetes has typically been referred to as "adult onset diabetes" there are now increasing numbers of overweight children being diagnosed with Type 2 diabetes. The treatment of this very preventable disease is one of the United States' top health care costs.

Remember that small changes can make a significant impact on your health. I have seen individuals substantially decrease their cholesterol and blood pressure with as little as a ten to fifteen pound reduction in their weight. As you become more aware of the lifestyle choices you have made which have contributed to your weight issues the more empowered you will be to make changes that will improve your health.

Even with your genetic factors that may predispose you to any one of these diseases, you are still in control. Do not use your family's health history as an excuse to throw up your hands and give in. Do not blame your genetics for your unsuccessful struggles with weight management. You can lay the groundwork of healthier eating choices and daily fitness habits to derail your genetic proclivities.

## Communicate with Your Doctor

Now you have a clearer idea of your risk factors. You are hopefully empowered to recognize that you do have control over your health. You *can* make a difference in the disease risk factors your genetics may predispose you to.

One of the most common goals I hear voiced by individuals who have decided to adopt a healthier lifestyle is to reduce or eliminate the medications they take. Although this is a worthwhile goal discuss it thoroughly with your doctor. Never, ever stop taking prescribed medications without guidance from your physician. As discussed, there are many genetic factors that have to be considered.

The safest plan is to inform your doctor that you are starting a healthier lifestyle approach to weight loss through more balanced eating and exercising. Inform him or her that you wish to reduce some of your prescription medications.

As your weight decreases, schedule follow-up visits with your doctor to discuss your prescriptions. Your physician should be supportive of your balanced goals and if not, find another physician.

## The Only Person You Can Change is *You*

*"Allow other people to own their own problems."*
*~Judy Bauman*

You have control over some of your surroundings. You have control over what you put in your mouth. You have control over the amount of time you commit to getting a little exercise in your day. But you do *not* have control over someone else.

If only we could all heed my Mom's wise advice, how much more peace would we have in our lives? I have spent so much time and energy trying to fix and change some of the people in my life over the years that I have completely neglected to take care of my own issues! No matter how much you want to, you cannot change someone else. Empowering yourself with this fact is an integral part of your weight management journey.

You may find that your family, parent, child, or spouse is the biggest saboteur in your life. If you are the only one in your life committed to making better choices, it will be challenging to change your lifestyle. You may even have to deal with people putting things in your path to trip over.

If you have made the decision to adopt some healthier habits then it is time to sit down and have a heart-to-heart with your family, friend, parent or child. This talk should be a time to express why *you* have decided to make these changes, why *you* feel this is the right time and why *you* need his or her support.

Hopefully, as I have often seen happen, the example you set and the rewards you experience will influence those around you. You may even inspire someone to adopt healthier changes too, but that will have to be their decision made in their own time. You do what *you* need to do and seek out people you can trust who will be there to support you.

## To Sum Up

Be encouraged as you learn from your past and move forward with brutal honesty and authenticity. What do you realistically have control over? What do you have in your power to change? The small, sustainable changes you make today will enhance the rest of your life.

**Chapter 5**

# Balancing Your Perspective about Your Weight

*"If you don't like something change it;*
*if you can't change it,*
*change the way you think about it."*
~ Mary Engelbreit, Artist and Illustrator

How important to you is the number that pops up on your bathroom scale? How much do you identify yourself with your body weight? Is your mood related to how well you stick to your *diet*? Do you find yourself imagining how much better your life would be if you were only thinner?

Yes, it is important to be a healthy weight, but it is *so* much more important to have a healthy image of yourself in spite of how much you weigh. Let's look at the truth about what your weight is and what your weight is not.

Your weight is...

- an indicator of your body's health
- something most people do have control over, whether you want to admit it or not
- influenced, to some degree, by your genetics

Your weight is not...

- a magic number that when attained will solve your life's other problems
- the key to true happiness in your life
- the answer to your self-esteem issues
- a reason to put off buying new clothes you would enjoy wearing and feel attractive in
- the cause of all your relationship problems

Do you identify with any of the latter statements? If so, it is time to work on gaining a new perspective. It will take time, but focusing more on your healthier image than a number on a scale will open you up to many possibilities.

Becoming consumed with a number can negatively dictate how you relate to almost everything else in your life. Are you aware of how your thinking is impacting your life right now? How many of us have put off truly living our lives because we have been waiting...waiting...waiting to weigh less?

## Get off the Scale

To many people's surprise, I *strongly* encourage my clients to stop weighing themselves every day. Daily weighing distracts from the reality that healthy weight loss takes time; a balanced goal is ½ to 2 pounds per week. Those amounts don't sound like much when you have a significant amount to lose, but note how the numbers add up over time:

**Long term results for a realistic goal of**
**~ ½ to 2 pounds of weight loss per week:**

| | |
|---|---|
| 1 month period | = 2 to 8 pounds |
| 3 month period | = 6 to 24 pounds |
| 6 month period | = 12 to 48 pounds |
| 12 month period | = 24 to 96 pounds |

Clearly, small changes over time really pay off. Be honest – would you be pleased with the benefits of a *permanent* weight loss of 10 or 12 pounds over the next few months? And yes, even ½ a pound per week is a success! This is a realistic and attainable goal when we begin adding small, healthier habits into our daily lives.

So, here is what it looks like in practical terms:

1.  First, weigh one time and *write it down* as you begin to incorporate a daily exercise routine and healthier eating choices then weigh again after 3 or 4 weeks. This may not sound like the advice you have heard in many programs, but it is the balanced approach.

2.  I then recommend you weigh yourself no more than once a week and *write it down.* Weighing more frequently will not show your progress and could get discouraging. Give your body time to change. Remember: You didn't gain the weight overnight so be patient.

3.  During the challenging holiday season from Thanksgiving through New Years and during vacations, I encourage my clients to focus on weight maintenance, not weight reduction. Again, this may sound surprising, but if you want a real-life approach to permanent weight maintenance, keep the big picture in mind.

    The holidays typically disrupt your normal routine. It may be tough to get in daily exercise when you are traveling, hosting friends and family, staying at someone else's home or eating out more than usual. My top two tips: Watch your portions closely and try to incorporate a daily walk with the family during the day or after a large meal.

4.  Finally, be patient and give yourself a break. Keep in mind that as you get older your body does change and your weight will likely fluctuate. Life transitions such as pregnancies, illness, surgeries, injuries, medications, divorce, tragic loss or dealing with depression also need to be taken into consideration as you set realistic, sustainable goals.

## Put the Emphasis Where it Belongs

Oprah Winfrey, media mogul, is known for many things, including her fluctuating weight. She has publicly shared over two decades of personal successes and mistakes along her weight management journey. We are in a nation where obesity has become an urgent problem, with one in five adults overweight and our children developing diseases related to obesity and inactivity. Oprah and her staff dedicated countless episodes of her television talk show to sharing other's stories and expertise about how to eat healthier and exercise more.

But it was Oprah's personal testimony during her 2010 interview with Barbara Walters that spoke to the heart of what realistic life change is all about: After acknowledging the importance of a balanced life she then shared, with resolve, that she will not be defined by her weight, that she will never diet again and that she refuses to beat herself up about it. She let it go.

It is time, as you strive for your own balance, to not only let go of the number on the scale, but to the power and energy you have placed into the mental battle with your weight.

Do not allow this battle to define you or hold you back any longer. Wouldn't the energy you expend trying to achieve that *ideal* weight be better used in another area of your life? Find the balance and let the ideal go. Stop beating yourself up about it and do what you can right now.

## How You Look and Feel

"Woo-wee, Girl, your cholesterol looks *fantastic!*"

You're not likely to hear this compliment from anyone but your physician. Truthfully most of us would rather hear, "Hey! You look great...have you lost weight?" Be honest – there is no denying we would like to feel attractive to ourselves and those around us. It also feels pretty good when your pants don't cut off the circulation to your lower legs when you sit down.

Although I consistently stress the importance of lifestyle change to improve your health and the things you and others don't see outwardly, there is nothing wrong with the desire to look better.

And although wanting to look better is great, be honest as you ask yourself if this has been your *only* reason for losing weight in the past. If so it may be the reason why you have chosen quick-fix, temporary methods. The balanced approach combines your desire to look better with the goal of improving your overall health to help you develop a healthier lifestyle.

## Why Do You Need and Want to Weigh Less?

Take a moment to write down your top five reasons to lose weight below. Use a pencil so you can erase and rewrite as you brainstorm.

Maybe, as we discussed, you'd like to reduce the amount of medications you are taking. How about that reunion coming up? Or do you want to have more energy, be more active and just feel better?

Whatever reasons you have, now is the time to be brutally honest with yourself.

1. _____
2. _____
3. _____
4. _____
5. _____

Reread your answers. Now, next to each statement write "want" or "need." Recognize that each of us distinguishes needs and wants differently. You may feel you *need* to lose weight for your upcoming reunion right now, but a more realistic need may be an immediate health concern.

Wants are not bad motivators either, but always remember that you're on a journey toward permanent change. Your wants can tempt you to seek short-term diets that will thwart your long-term goals, so keep those wants in perspective. I hope this review is enlightening to you.

## How Do You Perceive Your Weight?

Are you in denial about your weight?

Researchers from the Department of Preventive Medicine at Rush University in Chicago used data from a large study that tracked the risk of heart disease in young adults first recruited in 1985–1986. Over the course of the next 20 years, researchers tracked various statistical data about each participant such as height, body mass index, etc.

More importantly they surveyed what each participant perceived to be her body size as she pointed to a silhouette of a figure she thought most resembled her current size. Then she identified her ideal body size and the difference between the two.

What they found was very interesting. The obese women who perceived themselves accurately as overweight gained less weight annually than obese women who inaccurately identified themselves as a normal weight. The obese women whose ideal body size was "overweight" – in other words, neither slim nor obese – gained less weight annually than those whose ideal body size was a slimmer "normal weight."

Lead researcher Elizabeth Lynch, PhD noted:

"Our strongest finding was that obese women who perceive themselves to be much too big – which they are, from a medical perspective – maintain their weight better over time."

"Self-perception seems to be very important to weight maintenance," notes Lynch. "Obese women who face the fact that their bodies are much too large for optimal health are better at stopping weight gain and may even lose weight." She adds that size denial creates further weight problems probably because people in denial aren't able to start setting goals to change their behavior. (1)

## To Sum Up

Examine how much emphasis you place on your body weight. Make sure your desire to lose weight includes the goal of improved health and a clear understanding that permanent weight loss takes time and patience. Your perception of yourself matters – a lot. Balance your perspective and don't allow your weight to define who you are.

# Chapter 6

# SMART Goals

*"If you don't know where you are going,
you'll end up someplace else."*
*~ Yogi Berra*

Setting realistic goals and *writing them down* is an integral part of any lifestyle approach to weight management. For most individuals, the challenge is learning how to narrow down specific areas to focus on and then fine-tuning those goals into something realistic that can actually be achieved.

We are all familiar with the most popular New Year's resolution: "I'm going to lose weight." Is it any wonder so many give up this resolution after only a few weeks or months? A goal to "lose weight" is too broad and has no structure to support a commitment to new, healthier lifestyle habits.

Even stating the need to make some changes in your eating and exercise habits in order to reach a healthier weight range is not detailed enough. Use the following **SMART** Goal guide to assist you in your goal setting.

## Specific

Be as specific as possible. For example, let's focus on just one goal: Adding a daily exercise routine in order to reach a healthier weight, improve your health and reduce your stress. Begin by asking the questions:

- **Where** are you going to exercise? Would you be more likely to commit to a routine at home or do you need the structure and commitment to a local fitness facility? Maybe both?
- **Who** are you going to exercise with? Are you motivated to do it on your own or would you benefit from a friend or family member joining you for regular walks or sessions at the gym?
- **When** will you commit to exercising? Will you have to get up earlier in the morning to get on your treadmill because you know that once the day gets rolling there will be no time to stop to exercise? Will you stop by the gym at lunch or after work most days of the week?
- **What** are you going to do? What time of your day is best? What factors are in your control and which ones will be subject to your family's schedule or other commitments?

## Measurable

Is your new goal measurable? This is where you begin to ask the "how" questions and *write down* your progress.

- **How much** weight are you trying to realistically lose? A balanced starting goal is around 10% of your current body weight.
- **How many** times per week are you going to exercise? Three days at the gym and three days at home?
- **How many** minutes will you try to complete? If you're just starting an exercise routine, try 5 or 10 minutes and push yourself to do a little more each day.

## Achievable through Actions

Get detailed to achieve your goal. Lay out the action steps to achieve your goal. From setting your alarm clock at night for your morning exercise routine to adding the numbers of a few supportive friends into your cell phone, set yourself up for success and remove as many obstacles as possible.

## Realistic

Base your goals in reality. If you are in your 40's it is unlikely you will return to your teenage weight. Setting realistic goals will help you avoid failure down the road. Everyone's level of motivation, which will determine what you are willing to change or sacrifice for your goal, is different. What may seem realistic and reasonable to someone else may be completely unrealistic for you. That's okay. Ask yourself, do you know, and know that you know, that this goal can be reached? If you do, then great!

## Time-Based

Setting achievable goals requires a time-line. Be careful not to make the timeframe too long or you may set yourself up to procrastinate. Be just as careful to give yourself enough time to achieve each milestone toward your goal. A goal of losing between ½ to 2 pounds a week is balanced and typically attainable with small lifestyle changes.

Perhaps you don't currently eat breakfast, but you understand it is important for your health and metabolism to eat in the morning. As an example, put this into action by deciding on one or two foods you would be willing to eat in the morning – such as lowfat fruit yogurt or instant oatmeal – then add those to your grocery list. Go a step further and shop on Sunday afternoon so that your fridge and pantry are stocked at the beginning of the week with breakfasts ready to go.

# Pinpoint Where *You* Need to Change

Where do you identify on the spectrum of healthy lifestyle choices? I have provided two extremely simplified spectrum scales below for you to reference. One end of the spectrum reflects the individual who pays no attention to eating habits and is not physically active – the couch potato. The other reflects the athlete who exercises daily and is aware of every source of fuel that enters their body.

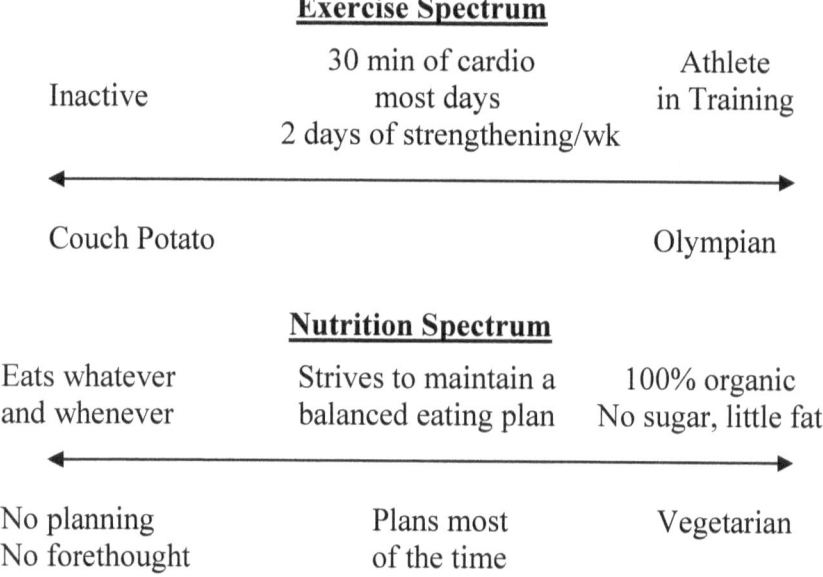

### Exercise Spectrum

|  | 30 min of cardio most days 2 days of strengthening/wk | Athlete in Training |
|---|---|---|
| Inactive |  |  |

⟵————————————————————⟶

| Couch Potato |  | Olympian |

### Nutrition Spectrum

| Eats whatever and whenever | Strives to maintain a balanced eating plan | 100% organic No sugar, little fat |
|---|---|---|

⟵————————————————————⟶

| No planning No forethought | Plans most of the time | Vegetarian |

Most of us fall somewhere in the middle and slide back and forth a little. That is okay. We may aim for five servings of fruits and vegetables daily plus a handful of minutes of exercise most days and hopefully *write down* and record some of our goals and choices on occasion to keep ourselves honest.

My hope, if you find yourself on the far left side of the exercise or nutrition spectrum, is that you have decided to make some changes to move a little bit more to the right. You don't have to be a professional athlete or a vegetarian to be healthy.

Ask yourself, today, what new habits you can create to move a little closer to the middle to be more balanced.

## Small Steps

Okay, so you have set some SMART goals for yourself, what is the next step? A term I use often is *baby steps*. Pick your most easily achievable new goal and start there. Guarantee a positive result in the very beginning by choosing something that you know you can achieve. Give it some time.

You have probably heard the saying that it takes 30 days to make or break a habit. That is especially true when it comes to adopting even small, balanced lifestyle goals. Please heed my advice to take it slowly.

Far too many zealous individuals, excited by the prospect of changing their lifestyle, attempt a clean sweep of *all* their unhealthy behaviors. They commit to a year-long gym membership, hire a personal trainer, resolve to become a vegetarian and burn all their fat pants on the front lawn. This type of radical change attempt is a sure recipe for failure and is sadly encouraged by far too many health professionals.

Remember your journey must be focused on balance and sustainability. This is not a sprint; it is a marathon that will last the rest of your life. But unlike a marathon, you won't have to wait until you cross the finish line to see the reward. You will reap all kinds of benefits along the way.

Take your time and give yourself a break. You will not achieve perfection – no one can. Be prepared for the reality that life is going to get in the way of your goals on occasion. When these times occur, don't give in. Revisit and revise your goals and jump back on track.

## Set Your Surroundings for Success

Help achieve your goals by changing your surroundings. Remember when your parents discouraged you from hanging around with the wrong group of kids because they knew their behaviors would eventually rub off on you? Consider this as you adopt a healthier lifestyle.

Try these two easy tips to improve your chances for success:

- Remove temptation from your home
  I will discuss this more in the chapter on Grocery Store Shopping, but I cannot stress enough how your home should be your safe haven for healthier food choices. If you know you are likely to reach for the junk food when you feel lonely, depressed, stressed or bored *do not* bring it in your home. Once the tempting foods are in your home it is much harder to resist the temptation to overindulge when the emotional urge or the "I deserve it," feeling strikes.

- Identify and Avoid Your Triggers
  What triggers your desire to overeat or skip your exercise session?
  I recently cut back on the amount of time I watch television. I simply came to a point where I realized that it was not a good use of my precious time. Also, I had reached a weight loss plateau and recognized that when I sat alone to watch TV I would inevitably grab something to eat and mindlessly munch away. The key word there is "mindlessly."

Take the time to identify areas in your life that serve as triggers to mindless eating or habits that you know are keeping you from being a healthier weight. Work on avoiding them when they arise.

## Group Support or On Your Own?

Having led behavior modification small groups I am a big proponent of a solid support system. I also support individuals who want to put the time and effort in to educating themselves about balanced eating, nutrition and fitness. There are many who do just that.

Everyone is different. There is no single program that will prove successful for everyone.

As previously mentioned, almost every community has numerous, affordable, balanced support groups. Even with the support of a group, be ready to accept responsibility for the choices you make in private. Being honest with *yourself* will still be the basis for any lifestyle change.

If you choose to go it on your own, do communicate with a few significant people in your life; a family member, friend or maybe an exercise buddy. Choose someone who will be there to encourage you and serve as a sounding board when you need it. The main key to doing it on your own is – you guessed it – *writing everything down.* Since you won't have anyone to be accountable to but yourself, be accountable to yourself!

Choosing to join a support group or local weight management program can be extremely beneficial. If you try one group and it doesn't seem to fit, try another.

Use the following guide to help you choose a balanced support group or program:

- Confidentiality
  You want to know that you can open up without group members blabbing your business to their family, friends or neighbors. A support group should be just that – supportive.

- Balanced nutrition and exercise education
  If the program does not include sound instruction and information to encourage smarter eating and consistent exercise – RUN!

- No required purchase of supplements or prepackaged meals
  Recognize what will inevitably happen when you stop taking the required supplements or foods. Do not join a diet group. You may be impressed with your initial, temporary results, but they will be just that – temporary.

- Equal emphasis on lowering your weight *and* maintaining a healthy weight range

Most participants lose weight when they join a program. Just as many gain it back if the program does not focus on adopting permanent lifestyle behaviors. Make sure any program or group you attend anticipates real life after the program has ended.

## To Sum Up

One of the main reasons so many weight loss attempts fail is because many focus on what everyone *else* is doing. Be honest with yourself and don't fall into this mindset. This is your personal journey and you're worth the time and effort to determine what will work in your daily life.

Adopting a new way of thinking, in addition to developing and writing down individual and specific goals, takes time. There is no quick fix when your overall goal is a healthier lifestyle. I would bet that you did not develop weight problems overnight, so please don't beat yourself up when you slip back into some of your old habits. As you experience the positive outcomes of your new habits, revise and refine your goals as you move forward.

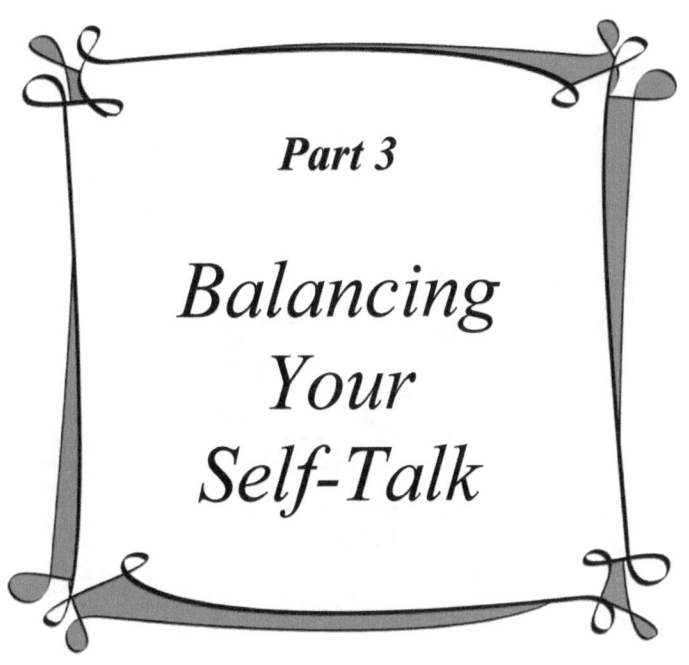

**Part 3**

# *Balancing Your Self-Talk*

# Chapter 7

# You're Talking to Yourself... and it's Okay

*"Every waking moment we talk to ourselves*
*about the things we experience.*
*Our self-talk, the thoughts we communicate to ourselves,*
*in turn control the way we feel and act."*
*~ John Lembo*

Do you consider yourself to be your friend? I know that is a strange question, but take a moment to think about it. Do you beat yourself up and insult your own efforts or do you reject negative, self-defeating statements? Do you look to others for approval, validation and acceptance or are you secure in yourself and your own decisions?

One of the best pieces of advice I received when I started my new life as a single mom was given to me by my wise friend, Sandra. She said, "When you are on an airplane, what is the first instruction the flight attendant gives in the event that the oxygen masks drop from overhead?" After giving me a moment to think about it she continued, "Put your *own* mask on before helping those around you."

Profound, isn't it? What good are you if you can't breathe? What good are you to others if you don't take care of yourself? Taking care of yourself will help you be a better parent, spouse, employee, volunteer or friend.

As the quote above reflects, inner communication will control the way you feel and act. When you stand undressed in front of a mirror – what are you thinking? What do you say to yourself when your doctor gives you the results of your blood work? When you can't fit into that pair of pants or shirt anymore, what do you think of yourself? What is your internal dialogue? Take a few moments to honestly think about this.

I want to again point out the obvious connection between your mind, body and spirit. Your internal dialogue will serve as a positive or negative force throughout your daily life. Begin to listen to what you are saying.

Take a moment to *write down* in your journal or in the spaces below the *first* thought that comes to your mind as you read the following statements silently:

- I can't fit into some of my favorite clothes anymore.
  Your self-talk's response:

  _____

  _____

- The doctor tells me I must make some changes or I will have to start taking medication for my heart or to regulate my blood sugar.
  Your self-talk's response:

  _____

  _____

- I really want to lose some weight and keep it off for good.
  Your self-talk's response:

  _____

  _____

Examine your first, inner response. I'm sure some of you feel sad when you realize that you would never say out loud to someone else the harsh words you have for yourself.

Sometimes, as you learn to listen to your self-talk, you may notice a continuing pattern of negativity. Maybe you are even starting to discover that *you* are your own worst enemy. This pattern can make or break a healthier lifestyle if you give way to defeating thoughts of powerlessness, lack of control and excuses.

Remember that we are typically the ones responsible for putting up barriers as we attempt to move forward.

As you wrote down your responses I hope you had some positive statements, too. *You* should be your biggest cheerleader. Your inner communication is the immediate source for encouragement and reassurance. Developing positive self-talk empowers you to make some tough changes and stick with them. Sure, it is helpful to have others around you, encouraging you, but the buck ultimately stops with you.

It is a rare person in our society, even one at a healthy weight, who feels genuinely satisfied with their body. Our culture puts an enormous emphasis on our outer appearance. Dr. Phil McGraw, psychologist, has shared an insight from his father that goes something like this: We wouldn't worry so much about what others thought of us if we realized how rarely they did. In other words, you should not focus on what others think of you because, in reality, they are not thinking about you – they are thinking about themselves.

That unbalanced focus makes us forget the blessings of good health and the gifts we should be sharing. It also removes your healthy self-love which will empower you as you move forward and become healthier. As you learn to listen to what you are saying to yourself notice any unconstructive, negative self-talk and nip it immediately. In time you can learn to replace it with encouragement and constructive tough love.

## Balanced Self-Love

A healthy dose of self-love and self-respect goes a long way to improving your behaviors. I find many of the individuals I work with don't value themselves very much. If you have not heard it lately let me be the one to tell you – you *are* valuable. Do you understand the importance of taking care of yourself in order to effectively care for those around you?

Begin with the understanding that balanced self-love will assist you in taking an honest look at who you are, right now, along your positive personal journey. Do you truly believe that you alone have what it takes to achieve your goals? Don't spend anymore of your precious time dwelling on the past or waiting for someone or something else to come along and fix what needs to be fixed. Think about it. You have everything you need.

Likewise, a balanced self-love opens the door to *receiving* healthy love and support from God and others. Although you have everything you need and are ultimately the one making the daily choices; seeking guidance, wise counsel, direction and assistance along the way makes the road *much* smoother. Accepting help when needed is a sign of strength, not weakness.

Be prepared to halt any comparison of yourself to someone else. Healthy self-respect empowers you with the understanding that comparing yourself to someone else, or attempting to change for someone else, serves no positive purpose.

Take some time to honestly reflect on your past weight loss attempts through the filter of healthy self-love. What was the main reason you wanted to weigh less? Did you want to lose the weight for someone else? Were you truly ready to adopt healthier, daily habits for a lifetime? An imbalance in this area is often the reason so many fail.

Developing healthy self-care, self-love and self-respect is life-changing. As you begin to foster these it may make all the difference as you commit to balanced, permanent changes in your everyday life.

## J.C.'s Inspiring Change

Many years ago I worked with a gentleman, J.C., who participated in my weight management program. J.C., a truck driver, had to weigh himself on the truck scales at work since our office scales only went up to 350 pounds. J.C. hung his head when he reported his weight at the beginning of our first session together – 485 pounds. He then explained why he was overweight.

"I drive a truck for a living so I'm always sitting down. I eat at truck stops and they only have unhealthy, greasy food. I don't have time to exercise because I'm driving so many hours." Even I felt bummed out after listening to all the negativity he had fed himself for years.

Although J.C. was taking a great first step by joining a balanced weight management program, he had convinced himself he was *powerless* in his weight struggle. He mentally placed barrier after barrier in front of himself.

I discussed the power of self-talk with J.C. and how becoming aware of what he said internally could make or break his lifestyle change. We examined his excuses and looked for the truth behind each of them.

Were all of his barriers truly beyond his control? Did he really have so few eating choices? Was there absolutely no time during the week for a little exercise?

J.C. and I chose small action steps for him to add into his daily routine. The exercise plan we decided upon involved simply walking from his front door to his mailbox and back as many times as he could. He began journaling what he was eating, how he felt and his self-talk, both positive and negative as his awareness grew. J.C. started taking a cooler in his truck cab filled with healthier snack options. We discussed portion size and smart meal options at truck stops.

I will never forget his appointment with me many months later when J.C. proudly reported that he had reached the 400 pound mark. We were both thrilled! He had adopted a new lifestyle that was paying off with great improvements in his health and self confidence.

I asked J.C. what difference that 85 pound loss had made in his life. He immediately responded: "I'm able to be intimate with my wife again and it's great!"

This answer surprised me. Not only had his health improved, but he was now able to see himself for the desirable guy he was, despite the numbers on the scale. This was an important milestone. J.C. was beginning to see that *he* was ultimately in control and understood that his improvements were going to keep him around longer for his family.

J.C.'s wife came to his next session. She was thrilled with his improved self-image, how he not only found himself attractive, but felt attracted to her again. His self-talk had drastically changed from the first time we met. He had begun to examine his excuses of powerlessness. He began to congratulate himself, to be proud of his accomplishments and develop positive self-talk that would allow him to continue to move forward. He was beginning to be his own best friend. We can all learn a lesson from J.C.

## Managing Your Stress

Stress happens. It is a part of life. Every single person handles stress a little differently and that means we each have a different way of using self-talk when dealing with stress. Making your health a priority coupled with the things you say in your own head are integral to managing stress.

We know stress can contribute to weight loss or weight gain, especially when it triggers emotional eating or lack of sleep. Even without that, a constantly hectic schedule with little time for planning or preparation will make it difficult to maintain a healthy lifestyle.

Some research indicates a link between obesity and stress. Recently there has been an increased discussion of an important hormone called cortisol, sometimes referred to as the "stress hormone."

Cortisol helps to maintain blood sugar levels and is released in excess during times of extreme physical or psychological stress. This can lead to an increase in appetite. Some studies have even shown that excess cortisol may be responsible for increased fat deposits around the abdomen. Increased fat around your belly increases your risk for heart disease.

But before you decide to blame cortisol for your weight issues, understand that everyone produces different amounts of cortisol. Weight is affected by many other factors, too, like your choices. Of course there are already companies who have jumped on the bandwagon to develop pills they claim will lower cortisol levels. Do not fall for it. Instead, incorporate the following strategies to better help you manage your stress:

- Exercise
  By far, the best method to help you reduce and manage your stress is with exercise. It is also the most effective method to reduce stress-induced cortisol levels. I have recently added what I refer to as my

"Forrest Gump Run" to my daily exercise routine. As I feel the pressure of things in life I have no power to change, I go out for a quick walk/run – maybe just 10 or 12 minutes. One of the most commonly reported benefits of exercise is better sleep which will also directly help you deal with life stresses.

- Get outside
Enjoying the outdoors and removing ourselves from the daily demands of our homes or offices has tremendous benefits. Take a walk after dinner or a drive in your car with the windows down. Make time to sit and watch the sunset or sunrise. Being in nature, even if just for a few minutes, aids your mind, body and spirit.

- Breathe
Take a moment to close your eyes, take a few slow, deep breaths and listen to the sound of the air flowing in and out of your lungs. Let your shoulders drop and slowly release the tension in each area of your body. A few minutes of relaxation techniques will decrease your blood pressure and your heart rate.

- Learn to let go
Many of us create stress for ourselves or adopt the stress of others. Recognize the role *you* have in creating some of the stress you are dealing with. Do you stress about something you have absolutely no control over? Identify these areas and issues and let them go.

- Learn to say, "No"
Establishing boundaries is an important part of a balanced, healthy lifestyle – especially for women. Why do we take on all that we do? If you feel overwhelmed with tasks and responsibilities, ask yourself why. Are you ultimately getting something from your choices – filling some place or need in

yourself that you don't know how else to fill? It's okay to say, "No." Make time to take care of yourself and don't feel guilty about it.

## To Sum Up

The things you say to yourself are incredibly powerful so make sure your self-talk is positive as you move forward on your journey. Here's the great news: The awareness you gain from paying attention to what you say to yourself will empower you. Learning to become your own best friend and respecting yourself will encourage you to look forward with balanced goals versus putting yourself down. Reevaluate your priorities and examine areas of your life that you can simplify in order to create more balance.

# Chapter 8

# Excuses

*"The best day of your life is the one on*
*which you decide your life is your own.*
*No apologies or excuses.*
*No one to lean on, rely on, or blame.*
*The gift is yours – it is an amazing journey –*
*and you alone are responsible for the quality of it.*
*This is the day your life really begins."*
*~ Bob Moawad, Author*

Who doesn't love a good excuse? We revel in pointing the finger at someone else for our condition, deflecting responsibility from ourselves. On my personal journey to find a healthy balance, I often used excuses to justify why I was still overweight.

Now is the time to honestly admit the role excuses have played in holding you back. The excuses we use to justify our weight are typically not valid. Determining what is truly in your control is a key to moving forward on your journey. Learn to take responsibility for your choices and evaluate your excuses as you proceed.

Begin to examine where your excuses are based. Have you ever worked up an alibi for your extra pounds before showing up to be weighed? How about when you have to go to a doctor's appointment? Do you come prepared with an excuse or two because you know your doctor will inevitably bring up the topic? Do you feel badly about it afterwards or even while formulating the excuse? Have you ever felt guilt from telling an outright lie regarding your weight? If you can relate with some of these thought processes, examine why you made that choice. Understand that valid excuses have no room for guilt, regret or embarrassment.

Many of us mistake excuses for truth which creates another barrier to progress. If you continue to make excuses, whether you say them to yourself or vocalize them to someone else, you will gradually begin to believe they are true.

It is hard to admit that our over-eating, under activity and excuse-making have led to our being overweight and unhealthy, but it is a necessary place to start. The journey to a lifetime of realistic, healthy weight management starts with this tough honesty.

Discover why you choose to make excuses. Look honestly at yourself as you examine these points.

## Why Do We Use Excuses?

***Reason #1*** *– It's not my fault. I can't help it.*

We, as humans, love to blame others for our problems. We want our issues to be someone else's fault. We want to point the finger at someone or something else because we don't want to face or accept the truth about our own choices.

Have you ever blamed a lifeless object for tempting you? "If the cake from my co-worker's party hadn't been so delicious, I wouldn't have had to have a second piece." Or, "A new fast food restaurant has opened on my street so it's too tempting not to stop by the drive-thru to pick something up while I'm making the long drive to and from work." How about, "I just can't help it."

Realistically you know the cake and the restaurant are not to blame for your weight problem. The cake did not force you to eat it and the restaurant did not make you stop your car at its drive-thru.

We try to convince ourselves that food, our upbringing, others around us, or even geographical locations are to blame for our weight. When we step back and listen to these statements, they sound ridiculous, don't they? We have in our control to help it, but we too often make an excuse instead of taking responsibility for our own choices.

Barring certain conditions which may require use of medications that may cause someone to gain weight, or an untreated food addiction, or unless you have been strapped to some type of surface and force-fed against your will, there is no one else to blame for how much you weigh. That is a hard one to accept, isn't it?

The only person who is ultimately responsible for your current weight is YOU. Where have you misplaced blame?

- Maybe you've blamed your parents for filling your home with high-fat junk foods while you were growing up.

- Maybe you've blamed the lunch ladies at your elementary school for their uncanny ability to deep fry okra and masterfully prepare irresistible frozen corndogs which led to your weight gain during adolescence.

- Maybe you've blamed your friends for encouraging you to eat out for lunch every day at work.

- Maybe you've blamed your partner in your old relationship who drove you to doughnuts to ease the loneliness, leaving you with regret that you did not purchase Krispy Kreme stock prior to the breakup.

- Maybe you've blamed your pet, because the dog food isle is opposite the candy isle at the grocery store.

- Maybe you've contemplated suing some major fast food restaurant because you're convinced you are the victim of their ingenious, brain washing marketing ploys – driving you to consume their high-fat, calorie laden, sugar-packed foods against your will.

Although some of these examples may be stretching it just a little, the reality is we often look for someone or something else to blame for our weight issues. It is hard to admit that we are the ones responsible for our current state. No more excuses – there is no one else to blame.

### *Reason #2 - Procrastination*

Why do we put it off? Waiting for some cosmic event to finally motivate us to improve our health does not make much sense, so why do we all do it? Procrastination is one of the main reasons why the weight loss industry earns an estimated $59.7 billion (yes, that is a B, as in BILLION) dollars for weight loss products and programs.

The National Center for Health Statistics estimates that two-thirds of Americans are overweight or obese. Again, this is often a gradual process with many of us asking, "How did I let this happen?" and "How can I get these pounds off now?"

Don't wait until your doctor says, "If you don't lose weight soon you are going to die," before deciding to take action. I am personally thrilled there are still doctors out there who are willing to cut to the core with some tough love. If you have heard this statement let it serve as an "ah-ha" moment and take action. Don't convince yourself that your weight is not a real concern.

### *Reason #3 – Excuses allow us to justify the unhealthy choices we don't want to give up and block us from adopting behaviors we know will take time and effort.*

I know you are familiar with the old saying, "Do what I say, not what I do." Who wants to give up the engrained, comfortable habits that feel so good? Although they may make you feel good for the moment, you know you dislike hearing about or dealing with the outcomes of your behaviors later.

Here is an example – If you know you have a hard time controlling your portion size of ice cream, why do you purchase a gallon of ice cream at the local grocery store and bring it into your home? You have immediately set yourself up for failure. Then, when the kids ask, over the empty tub, "Hey, where is the ice cream?" your response is a quick excuse or defense.

Yes, it can be challenging to find time to exercise every day. Yes, although healthy food is delicious, it is not the same as your current daily fast food run. There are dozens of excuses to support why you can't exercise and eat healthier, but you know there are a hundred reasons why you *should* choose moderate exercise and healthier food choices on a regular basis.

*Reason #4 – Making excuses takes your power away.*

Feeling completely powerless to handle a situation or solve a problem can lead to a load of excuse making.

Some feel that admitting they need some help or admitting they have a problem demonstrates a lack of power, but in truth, it is completely the opposite. Accepting that you have a problem demonstrates how much genuine power you have.

Many of us feel we are powerless to lose weight and even more powerless to maintain a healthy weight. Are you giving away your power because you want someone else to fix it for you?

Beliefs that you're just not strong enough, not committed enough or that someone else is more educated about it than you are all compound the negative feeling of powerlessness. There are countless supplements and pills on the store shelves produced for the sole purpose of making a buck off of millions who feel they can't possibly do it on their own.

Do not fool yourself. Yes, I said "fool *yourself.*" That particular weight loss pill manufacturer did not force you to buy their product, but they rely on your feeling of powerlessness to make their money. The fast food restaurant did not force you to walk in their door and purchase those unhealthy items, but they know the fat, sugar and salt are strong lures to bring you back in.

Contrary to popular belief, there is no battle between a little devil on one of your shoulders and an angel on the other while you stroll down the aisles of your neighborhood grocery store. Do not excuse your behavior by adopting the role of victim.

## Identify Your Excuses

Here is another opportunity to be honest with yourself. In the space below, or in your journal, *write down* the top five excuses you have held on to. They may be related to your upbringing, your family, your dislike of exercise or any number of other factors.

1. _____

2. _____

3. _____

4. _____

5. _____

Now recognize how these statements and attitudes have held you back. Remember: YOU hold all the cards when it comes to your health. It is time to stop pointing the finger and take responsibility.

## To Sum Up

You may desperately want your unfounded excuses to support your unhealthy habits, but they will never hold water. As you continue forward on your journey be keenly aware of excuses. *You* are in control of your weight. Your weight is not in control of you.

**Chapter 9**

# Learning from Laughter
# and Tough Love

*"You grow up the day you have your first
real laugh at yourself."*
*~ Ethel Barrymore, Actress*

Learning to laugh at our bizarre thinking and excuse making about weight issues can be a healthy thing. Jeff Foxworthy's *"You Might Be a Redneck If..."* jokes are hilarious. Many people are surprised that Southerners are not offended by them. Why? Because the jokes are, for the most part, based in truth.

In order to help us along our honest path of reality-based weight management I have created my own *You Might Be* list below. As you might guess, many of these have been drawn from my own life experience. Others are from a few of the hundreds of amazing people I have had the pleasure to guide who have helped me along my personal journey.

- If you know intellectually what a *belt* is, but can't recall the last time you personally owned one, let alone wore one...you might have a weight problem.

- If two local fish camp restaurants had to close down when you went on your last diet...you might have a weight problem.

- If your order at the local fast food restaurant consists of a triple cheeseburger and mega-size fries, followed by, "A small diet soda please…I'm trying to watch my calories,"…you might have a weight problem.

- If you cannot recall the last time you shopped on the skinnier side of *Dress Barn*…you might have a weight problem.

- If that "plant stand," "clothes hanger" or "storage platform" in your living room was originally a piece of exercise equipment…you might have a weight problem.

- If you tell people you are still carrying around your baby weight and your kids are in their teens or twenties…you might have a weight problem.

- If you go out of your way to travel to a grocery or convenience store where you will not be recognized…you might have a weight problem.

- If the main reason you purchase a car with a hatchback is to have the clearance to throw an impulse buy from the grocery bags in the back of the car into the front passenger seat…you might have a weight problem.

- If you have attempted a diet with only one food item in the title such as "grapefruit," "hotdog" or "cabbage soup"…you might have a weight problem.

- If you've ever thrown something in the trash after mustering the willpower not to eat it, only to go back later, dig it out of the trash and scarf it down…you might have a weight problem.

- If you've ever asked your children to put something from the buffet line on *their* plate for you to eat…you might have a weight problem.

- If you refuse to eat at a restaurant unless the menu includes the phrases, "All you can eat" or "Endless buffet"...you might have a weight problem.

- If, as you hear a skinny person express, "Oh, I just can't gain weight...it doesn't matter how much or what I eat," you feel your jaw clinching, your eye twitching and envision their slow, painful death...you might have a weight problem.

- If you've ever *eaten* a skinny person who has expressed the same...you might have a weight problem.

- If every piece of clothing you purchase has to have *at least* one *X* on the label...you might have a weight problem.

- If your closet has enough elastic to weave a small, circus safety net...you might have a weight problem.

- If you shop at *Big and Tall*, but you're not tall...you might have a weight problem.

- If, during an acceptance speech, you feel the need to thank your friends *Sara Lee*, *Little Debbie* and *Ben and Jerry* for the person you are today...you might have a weight problem.

- If your doctor credits you for his summer beach home...you might have a weight problem.

- If you begin most meals with the statement, "I'll start my diet Monday morning,"...you might have a weight problem.

Learn to laugh at yourself and remember that you are not alone.

## Tough Love

> *"You may not realize it when it happens, but a kick in the teeth may be the best thing in the world for you."*
> *~ Walt Disney*

Now for the tough love. Yes, it is beneficial to laugh at ourselves and to realize we are not alone. It is just as important on your journey to realize when your weight, or the weight of someone you care for, is reason for concern.

Remaining in denial could mean the difference between life and death. I hope, by now, you have seriously considered the consequences of what the excess weight you are carrying will do for your health, your self-esteem and your future. It is time to hold yourself accountable.

Maybe you picked up this book for a friend, relative or teenager whose weight causes you to worry about their health. How do you go to someone you love and express your concern about their weight and health? Badgering and nagging someone has never proven to be a successful method of persuasion, in fact it can make the situation worse.

The best choice is to sit your loved one down and express sincerely your concern and ask if there is something you can do to help. The choice to adopt a healthier lifestyle and lose weight must come from *their* desire to make a change, not *your* desire for them to change. You cannot force someone to lose weight, but you can express your genuine love and support for them. Encourage healthy behavior when you witness it, especially among kids. Set a good example with your own choices.

## Parents – Accept Responsibility

In my desire to help you honestly examine yourself, I would like to take a moment to address parents. In my lifetime, I have never witnessed a child drive themselves to a grocery store to shop for food to stock their fridge or pantry. Nor have I witnessed a kid pulling a car up to the drive-thru window.

You, as a parent, must take responsibility for the food you allow in your home, your choice of restaurants and the food choices your children make on a daily basis. Setting the groundwork for a healthy adult begins in childhood with a focus on balance and smarter choices.

Here is a reality check – about two thirds of overweight kids will become overweight adults. The key again is balance. There is no reason you can't enjoy a meal out, even a fast food meal occasionally, but that cannot be the norm.

Parents also have a responsibility to teach and guide their children to accept who they are – no matter what their size or shape.

Let's face it, we live in a looks-obsessed society where unrealistic media images surround our children every minute of the day. I have worked with kids and teens whose parents have so impressed on them a distorted body image and unhealthy relationship with food, that I believe it borders on child abuse.

I have witnessed parents, embarrassed by how their children look, hounding them to lose weight so they can conform to what "everyone else" looks like. On the other extreme, kids with completely disengaged parents, who grow up surrounded by junk food and soft drinks, spending hours in front of the TV, computer and various gaming devices will have a difficult road ahead. Do not initiate your kids early into a lifelong struggle with weight and health issues.

If you, as a parent, can identify with either one of these scenarios please take a moment to examine your own motives. Your main goal should be to encourage healthier eating and exercise by setting the right example *first*. Use these tips to assist you as you create a healthy environment for your family:

- Keep fruits and vegetables stocked at home and encourage your kids to eat them daily.
  Include the fresh items your family likes on your weekly store list. Designate a large bowl in plain view and keep it filled with bananas, apples or other fruits.

- Remove unhealthy food from the home.
  It is fine to enjoy some treats once in a while, but make it a rare occasion, not something they can grab

on a daily basis. This especially applies to soft drinks and junk foods that provide no nutritional value.

Soft drinks are simply liquid desserts so don't bring them in your home. Many grocery stores are offering healthier snack alternatives which have reduced sugar and have eliminated the transfats. If you are in a habit of reaching for unhealthy snacks, begin by substituting a healthier choice for one of your daily items. The more often you choose the healthier option the more you will become accustomed to it.

- Set time limits on screen and phone time for your kids.
  TV, computers, gaming devices, cell phones, etc. should have a daily limit. Also, collect the devices at a determined time at night so your child can get adequate sleep. I understand the commitment this takes for you parents as I live it daily. Your personal example will go a long way in helping to set balanced boundaries.

- Take your kids outside to play.
  Kids need some encouragement to get more active and play outside. Understandably, security issues are a concern so you need to be prepared to go outside and play too if the situation warrants. Your child learns from your example, and naturally craves undivided time with you, so make active time a priority.

## To Sum Up

You are not alone in much of your thinking or in many of your past, unbalanced attempts to lose weight. Move forward with laughter and tough love. There are times for both along your journey to a balanced, healthier lifestyle. Parents, love your children.

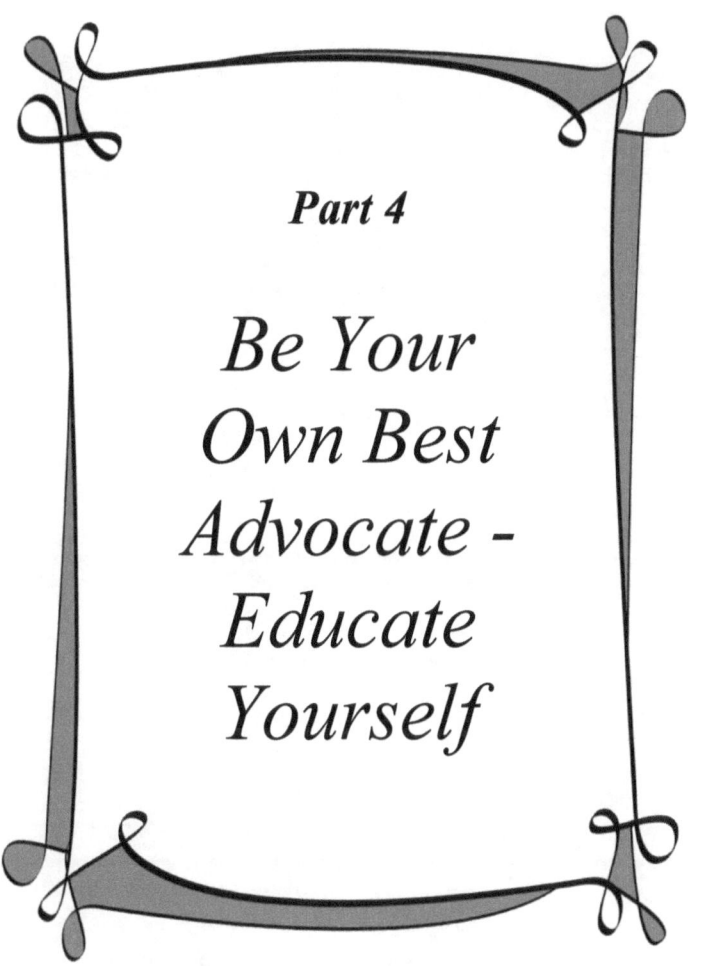

*Part 4*

*Be Your
Own Best
Advocate -
Educate
Yourself*

# Chapter 10

# The Truth Behind What You *Think* is the Truth

*"The ugly truth is always better
than the best-dressed lie."*
*~ Ann Landers*

By now you have examined your inner dialogue and assessed your personal and family health risk factors. Hopefully you have decided to stop making excuses and are ready to commit to improving your health. Where do you go from here?

One of the most wonderful "things" in life you have control over is what you choose to believe. So start there.

Have you ever heard the saying, "Don't believe everything you hear and only half of what you see?" Sadly, we have given away much of our ability to make good choices, in part because dieting and weight-loss advertisers are such geniuses at packaging half-truths in attractive wrappings. With that in mind, I encourage you to research for yourself what I will share with you in this chapter. As you continue on your honest path, keep your mind open for more truth.

## Doctors and Nutrition

I advise anyone I work with to share with their doctor the steps they are taking to adopt a balanced, healthier lifestyle. But, I do not typically advise clients to consult their doctor about healthy eating and exercise guidelines unless that doctor has training in this area.

Instead I recommend my clients make an appointment with a local Registered Dietician whose sole purpose is to help them adopt healthier eating habits.

For exercise, I recommend a certified personal trainer at a reputable establishment. By "reputable" I mean one that requires its specialists to have degrees in their field and/or completed certifications and ongoing continuing education. Make sure your journey to a healthier lifestyle is guided by others who have the training to back up what they are teaching you.

Just because the trainer at the gym looks fit does not mean you should take his or her nutrition advice. Adopt the same standards as you choose your personal physician. Do not assume that because someone has a medical degree they know more about healthy eating and exercise than you do.

I believe the vast majority of doctors want what is best for their patients. The few who show up on TV promoting potentially dangerous supplements or weight loss pills with proven serious side-effects are not the norm. They are being paid for their endorsement.

There are plenty of honest physicians who have educated themselves about balanced healthier lifestyles, but it is still the rare doctor who focuses on disease prevention. Conventional medicine is still largely based on the premise of treating sick people.

You must determine if you and your primary care physician see eye-to-eye about a healthy lifestyle. A caring physician will take the time to answer your questions. I have had some intense debates with physicians regarding various diets and supplements they prescribe.

One doctor in particular was encouraging *all* of his overweight patients to attempt an unbalanced, high-protein, very, very low-carbohydrate diet which was experiencing a resurgence in popularity. I asked him how he could prescribe this for his patients when he knew just how risky this high-fat, low carbohydrate diet could be. He shrugged his shoulders and replied, "Hey, they'll lose some weight."

Is it surprising to learn that doctors in our country rarely complete the recommended 25 hours of nutrition education during their entire degree tenure? A recent study from the University of North Carolina reported that U.S. medical schools are actually providing fewer nutrition education hours now than they were six years earlier. (1)

With the growing trend of obesity in our country one would assume that our medical schools would put *more* of an emphasis on teaching our front-line health providers the proven correlation between good nutrition and health.

Educate yourself and find a doctor who is interested in encouraging you to adopt a healthier lifestyle. You know your body better than anyone else so stand up for yourself.

## The Balanced Way to Lose Weight

Whether from fasting and juice cleanses, prepackaged reduced calorie meals or dieting and exercise, when you eat and drink fewer calories than your body is using you will lose weight. This is simply how the human body works. It is up to you to educate yourself to choose the healthiest, long-term approach.

The best and balanced path to reducing your weight will have these components:

- Eat Less and Eat Smarter
  Real life should include a variety of real foods just a little less of them. Limit the processed foods and make smarter choices overall about what you are using to fuel your body. Educate yourself or seek advice from a registered dietician or sound support group about how to buy and prepare foods. Learn how to make healthier choices when you eat out. The key component is eating and drinking fewer calories than your body is using in the day.
  **FACT**: A reduction of 500 calories per day will equate to the balanced ½ to 2 pounds of weight loss per week for most individuals.

- Exercise
  Understanding the health benefits alone should be enough to prompt you to find new ways to increase your activity and move more every day. When you

lose weight you don't lose just fat, you lose weight from all areas of your body. You want to maintain as much of your lean muscle as possible as your weight decreases, so eating smarter and exercising must go hand-in-hand. Consistent, daily exercise must become as essential to your day as eating when it comes to weight maintenance.

- Get Your Sleep
  We are learning more and more about the connection between lack of sleep and the negative effects it has on the body, especially related to weight gain. When your goal is a healthier weight range it is essential to get the right quality and quantity of consistent sleep. You need seven to nine consecutive hours of sleep every night.

- Patience
  I cannot stress enough the importance of having patience while you adopt a healthier lifestyle. Your deeply-ingrained eating habits will take time to change. Your misconceptions about dieting and weight loss may take some time to let go. Give it time and give yourself a break. Most of us gained our excess body weight over time and it will take time to lose it. Balanced eating and exercise do not require perfection because perfection can never be achieved.

## Spot Reduction

If I had a dollar for every time someone has asked me, while grabbing and shaking some area of their body with one or both hands, "Gretchen, how can I get rid of this?" I would be a very wealthy woman indeed. I always love this question. Why? Because spot reduction is one of the biggest myths out there and I thrive on opportunities to share the truth about myths that waste so much of people's money.

Side note: If your personal trainer is encouraging you to do some exercise to shrink a specific area of your body – like your stomach or the back of your upper arms – I strongly recommend you get a new trainer.

Now, back to the spot reduction myth: You cannot reduce fat in one specific area of your body.

I do inform my clients that they can achieve their desired result by either paying for liposuction to actually remove the fat cells, or they can have patience, while they strengthen and tone their whole body, and learn to delight in and accept their own body, fat pockets and all.

Yes, we all have areas of fat we would like to remove from our bodies. Again, this is greatly determined by our genetics, pregnancies, the aging process and other factors.

The misinformation flowing through the airwaves continually surprises me. I shake my head at the exercise equipment infomercials that promise to give you those "6-pack abs." The most hilarious thing about that phrase is that the 6-pack may have helped cause your abdominal weight problem in the first place. Am I right?

Bottom line about infomercial spot-reduction claims: It will not matter how many times you rock back and forth or side-to-side. Unless you are actually the model who is demonstrating the exercise, you will never, *ever* have his or her abdominal muscles. Those models were hired for the way their abdominal muscles *already looked*, not because they achieved those results using that piece of equipment.

Some equipment users will disagree, claiming that they did lose weight and toned their (fill in the blank). My challenge is always: Did you lose weight ONLY in that specific area? I have yet to see a 300 pound man walking around with ripped abdominal muscles while the rest of his body remains unchanged. That is not how our bodies work.

What individuals typically experience is weight loss from head to toe. I will discuss this further in the section on *Balanced Exercise*. Do not just take my word for it. Research this on your own to help you understand that you cannot just reduce one, specific area. In fact, the one "problem" area you want to reduce the most may be the last place to see a significant reduction because of the concentration of fat cells in that area.

With that being said, however, let me clarify that I am not opposed to exercise equipment purchased from infomercials in general. If you enjoy using your abdominal cruncher, twister, stepper, whatever – that is great! By using that piece of equipment consistently and increasing your heart rate enough to break a sweat, you are exercising and that is all that matters.

## I Want to Lose *Just* Fat

No matter how much we wish it or how "fast and easy" the claims of that $19.95 supplement sound, when you lose weight you cannot lose *just* fat.

As you lose weight it is imperative to exercise in order to maintain as much muscle mass as possible. You may know or have seen someone who has lost a significant amount of weight by only cutting back on their eating, or having a surgical procedure. The physical results are not always that desirable.

The weight loss "reality" shows on television are a good example of why it is important to exercise in combination with a reduced calorie plan. Of course the weight lost on those shows is highly unrealistic for the average individual. Those participants are pushed to lose as much as 15 pounds or more in a week and are monitored closely by physicians and other professionals.

No pill or supplement can replace a balanced exercise routine.

## "I Have a Slow Metabolism"

A frequent comment I hear, especially from those lugging around lifelong dieting baggage is, "I have a slow metabolism." Notice this is in the form of a resolved statement, not a question. I immediately reply, "How do you know?" The answer I typically get is not an answer at all, but rather a list of reasons why the person is unable to lose weight.

The truth is the vast majority of us do not have anything out of whack with our metabolism. This is as disheartening for me as it is for you. The "metabolism excuse" was one of *my* personal favorites to justify being overweight. It just sounds good, doesn't it?

Realistically, a slow metabolism is rarely the cause of weight gain or the inability to lose weight. A change in your weight is typically related to the amount of calories you are taking in versus what you are expending, as discussed earlier.

What is your metabolism? Basically, metabolism is your body's way of combining the nutrients (food and beverages) and oxygen in your body to release the energy it needs to function. This is measured in kilocalories, commonly referred to as calories. A calorie is a unit of energy. I will discuss calories and nutrition in more detail later. There are three main types of metabolic rates:

1. Resting Calories – Resting Metabolic Rate (RMR) or Basal Metabolic Rate (BMR)
   This is the rate at which your body uses energy to keep your basic functions going – breathing, circulation, cell repair – *while you're at rest*. Most people are surprised to learn that our RMR uses about 60% to 75% of our energy for these basic, automatic bodily functions. This percentage does not take into account the energy needed for your daily activities or exercise routine.

2. Processing Food - Thermogenesis
   Digesting, absorbing, transporting and storing the food and beverage you consume accounts for about 10% of the calories used during your day.

3. Exercise and Activity Calories
   The remaining percentage applies to the calories you burn during your daily activities and planned exercise routine, aggressive vacuuming, pushing the mower around the yard, etc.

The sum of these three equals your Total Metabolic Rate (TMR).

# The Importance of Muscle

Your metabolism can be affected by your genetics, but one of the most important factors determining your metabolic rate is the amount of muscle you have. Muscle simply requires more energy to operate so the more muscle you have the higher your metabolism rate and the more calories you burn, even at rest.

Men have the advantage because they have higher muscle mass than women. But as we get older we all typically lose muscle mass. This also explains why our metabolism slows down slightly as we age. The good news is that you can build more muscle at any age to aid in increasing your metabolism.

Your metabolism may also slow down if you choose not to eat enough. Many people are often surprised to hear me say, "You have got to eat to lose weight." But it's true. If you regularly skip meals your body will begin to pull not only from fat stores to gain energy, but from the lean tissue of your body as well. Sure, you may lose weight by not eating, but at what cost to your muscle mass?

What about the popular misconception that someone's metabolism can be irreparably damaged by yo-yo dieting – losing and gaining weight over and over? For the majority of former yo-yo dieters this is not the case. Depending on how much weight a person has lost and gained during these cycles, he or she may have reduced muscle mass, but that muscle can be regained over time through daily exercise and modest strength training sessions.

The only way to determine if you actually have a slow metabolism is to be tested for it.

In the past, tests were cumbersome, expensive and had to be conducted in research facilities. Researchers placed subjects in atmospherically controlled chambers and measured the exact amount of heat released from the subject's body at rest. That process determined one's "direct calorimetry." Or researchers used "indirect calorimetry," in which a subject or patient fasted overnight and researchers captured their subject's exhaled gases in plastic bags to determine the ratio of gases. This in turn would reveal their metabolic rate. Most of us don't have the time or funds to complete testing like this.

Today there is a hand-held device approved by the FDA that analyzes a person's exhaled gases and calculates the metabolic rate. Many qualified exercise facilities, wellness centers, spas and local universities are offering this service for a relatively moderate fee. If you feel it is necessary or you are simply curious, then go ahead and have your metabolism tested. You can then, once and for all, determine if you indeed have a slow metabolism or if you have used it as an excuse and a barrier to moving forward.

For the rest of us who are ready to move forward, there are things you can do to maintain a healthy metabolism.

- Exercise
  Consistent, moderate, daily exercise including two or three days of strength training per week helps maintain muscle mass. Remember, the more muscle you have, the more calories you burn, even at rest.

- Eat Regularly
  Do not skip meals. If you do not currently eat breakfast, make that one of your first goals. Eat when you are hungry and keep healthy snacks on hand.

- Get Your Fruits and Veggies
  Eat at least 3 servings of vegetables and 2 or 3 servings of fruit per day, preferably whole fruit and raw or steamed vegetables to maintain most of their vitamins and minerals.

If you are following all of these guidelines and are *still* unable to lose weight, schedule an appointment with your doctor. There are some medical conditions, such as an underactive thyroid, that may inhibit your ability to lose weight.

## Vitamin and Mineral Supplements

Supplementation is an often confusing and misunderstood topic. Because of this many avoid taking vitamins and minerals because they are not only unsure of what to take, but fear doing more harm than good. This thinking is understandable. There are so many brands and combinations offered in advertisements and on store shelves, that how does one choose? I hope the following Q & A serves to clarify some of these points.

Q. Should I take a vitamin and/or mineral supplement?

A. Everyone, in my opinion, should be taking a daily multivitamin.
Supplements *do not* and *cannot* replace a variety of healthy foods in your diet and will not make up for a lack of good nutrition. This is why they are called *supplements*. But because it is difficult to get all of the nutrients we need every day, we can look at a balanced multivitamin as a back-up or insurance policy.

Speak to your physician to make sure your supplement will not interfere with prescriptions you are currently taking.

Take your multivitamin once a day with a meal or divide it and take half with breakfast and half with dinner in order to aid in its absorption.

A good multivitamin will have these basic components:

- Water soluble vitamins, meaning they dissolve in water, like Vitamin C and the B's: thiamine (B1), riboflavin (B2), niacin, pantothenic acid, B6, biotin, folic acid, and B12. Most of these vitamins are not stored in the cells and pass out of the body quite easily so they need to be replenished every day. Vitamin C is essential for your immune system so you should focus on eating foods rich in Vitamin C. The B vitamins assist in the conversion of food to energy, keep your cardiovascular system healthy and help your body handle stress.

- Fat soluble vitamins A, D, E and K. These vitamins dissolve in fat, store in the cells of the body and do not pass as easily as water soluble vitamins.

- Minerals. Calcium, zinc, potassium, iron, magnesium, phosphorus, and selenium assist in the body's growth and help it function optimally.

- Additional antioxidants are a welcome addition to the common multivitamin. Antioxidants may protect our cells from damage to slow or prevent the development of cancer. Lutein, which gives fruits and vegetables their yellow color, is good for eye and heart health. Lycopene, which gives fruits and vegetables their red color, is good for prevention of certain cancers, eye and heart health.

Q. How much of each vitamin and mineral do I need? Is it possible to take too much?

A. Just because something is good for you *does not* mean you should take too much. Look for a multivitamin that provides approximately 100% of the daily value (DV). Remember that many breakfast cereals and cereal bars are fortified with vitamins and minerals too so read your labels and be aware of how much you are taking in.

Your body gets rid of excess water soluble vitamins like C and the B vitamins when you pee. This is typically why your urine is darker after taking your multivitamin. Your body will take what it can use and dispose of what it doesn't.

Fat soluble vitamins like A, D, E and K are stored in the cells of the body. Vitamin D may protect from osteoporosis, high blood pressure, cancer, and several autoimmune diseases, but in excess can cause kidney damage. It also assists in the body's absorption of calcium, but taking too much vitamin D will actually cause calcium to leach from the bones. Taking too much calcium is not healthy either as it may cause kidney stones.

Q. Should I take an extra, specific vitamin on top of my multivitamin?

A. If you are eating a variety of nutrient-dense foods it is highly unlikely that you need to take additional supplementation above the 100% DV. If you suspect a vitamin or mineral deficiency speak with your doctor or registered dietician. Remember that many of the packaged foods we eat are also fortified with vitamins and minerals.

Premenopausal women may benefit from a multivitamin that offers a little more iron. Post menopausal women, due to the increased risk of osteoporosis, may benefit from an additional calcium supplement if they don't drink milk or eat yogurt or cheese. Again, do your own research and choose wisely.

Q. Organic supplements or man-made? Is one absorbed better than the other?

A. Organic vitamins and minerals are more potent and are more readily absorbed by the body. Synthetic supplements are going to be less expensive, but organic will give you more benefit for the investment. Whether you choose man-made or organic, make sure your multivitamin does not have additives like sugar, yeast, salt, gluten, or unnatural fillers, colors, or preservatives.

## Protein Supplementation

Once again I come to a sensitive subject. There are some active people, typically men, who are passionate about the topic of protein supplementation. These gentlemen believe with their whole heart that the results they are achieving in the gym are due in some part to the expensive protein supplement they consume daily.

I have to admire the marketing savvy of this billion dollar supplement industry. Its promoters have successfully convinced untold thousands of teenagers and adults that they need to purchase their products in order to achieve increased muscle mass.

Here is the truth – The only way to build more muscle is by lifting more weights. There is no need to supplement with protein shakes, pills or powders. The products you are purchasing are not readily absorbed by the human body and are a waste of money.

It is true that you need to eat more and add some more protein in your day when you are exercising intensely. Your body will be able to utilize another chicken breast, a couple more eggs and another glass of milk much more than a supplement. If you are one of the individuals I am speaking of, I encourage you not to take my word for it, but to do the research on your own. Do not take the word of the company selling you the product as they do have an agenda.

## I'm Big Boned So I'll Always Be Overweight

"I've always worn a larger size than everyone else my height."
"Even when I eat healthier and exercise I still can't get my weight down to where it is supposed to be on the weight charts."

Bottom line: That's okay. You may have a larger bone structure than someone else, but don't use that as a justification for being overweight. We all vary in shapes and sizes. Simple logic will tell you that the taller you are, the larger your frame and therefore the more you can weigh.

If you have found, with consistent healthy eating habits and daily exercise, that you can't reach the recommended weight range on the charts for your height, then it is time to learn to be happy with *your* healthiest weight.

Let go of any thoughts or excuses that have held you back from a healthy appreciation of your own body.

## To Sum Up

Education is power. Research for yourself before accepting what advertisers are pushing or the crowd is adopting. Strive to eat a variety of healthy foods and supplement with a daily, organic multivitamin with a meal. Most importantly, appreciate the body you have been given.

# Chapter 11

# Discovering Your Own
# Balanced Weight Range

*Become the expert of your own body.*

One of the most valuable choices you can make is to take responsibility for your own health.

Dr. Mehmet Oz, surgeon and nationally syndicated health advocate, encourages all of us that we are the experts of our own bodies. Think about it. No other human knows your mind, body and spirit better than you do.

Your journey will lead you to *become* the expert of your own body. How? By taking the time to acknowledge where you are right now, examine your family history, evaluate your past attempts to lose weight and empower yourself through education to let go of old baggage and misinformation. All of these steps advance you toward gaining a better understanding of the control you have over your health and your choices.

As you accept responsibility for your health you will learn to appreciate how unique you are as an individual. We are all different. There is no cookie-cutter solution for everyone. Empowered with this knowledge you won't have to rely on your doctors, your family, your friends and *especially not* the images in most diet advertisements to tell you the exact number that should pop up on *your* bathroom scale. Take my advice and guidance with that of others and use that information to assist you in making your own decisions.

# 135 Pounds or BUST!

Let's begin with a balanced and honest approach. How realistic is it that someone could maintain one exact number for their weight over the long-term? It isn't. This is yet another reason why so many become discouraged and eventually give up along the way. Your weight and your body are *guaranteed* to change during your lifetime.

Instead of choosing one, unrealistic number on the scale, begin by considering this question – what is a healthy *range* for your weight? A fixation on an ideal will set you up for continual disappointment, especially if you have never come close to reaching that ideal. There are many, many factors that go into determining an individual's healthy weight range. It takes some investigating. I promise it will be well worth your time to educate yourself about your own, wonderful body. There is no magic weight number for you, but there are tools and guides that will help you determine a healthy weight *range*.

I have included information about three helpful tools that will assist in determining your individualized healthier weight range. Be prepared as it may be drastically different than what you have thought in the past due to misinformation. Use these tools to help you take control of your health and develop realistic goals for yourself. Taking the time to gather this information will empower you as you move forward.

## #1: Body Mass Index

Body Mass Index or BMI is a measure of someone's weight in relation to their height. Some dismiss this guide because it only takes into consideration someone's height and weight, but it is a good tool to assist you in determining a healthy weight range and one that is widely used within the medical profession.

An individual is clinically defined as obese when their Body Mass Index is 30 or higher. Various studies continue to show that a BMI over 30 is associated with increased disease risks. Health professionals consider that a BMI of 25 and below reflects a healthier weight.

The following Body Mass Index chart is one you may have seen in your doctor's office or possibly attached to some of your health or life insurance forms. Insurance companies use this calculation to determine your individual disease risk, along with genetic factors and past medical history.

Take some time to study this chart. Determine where your weight currently registers and what a healthier range may be. Remember, this is just one tool to consider as you educate yourself and determine your healthy weight range.

## Body Mass Index

| Height | 19 | 20 | 21 | 22 | 23 | 24 | 25 | 26 | 27 | 28 | 29 | 30 | 31 | 32 | 33 | 34 | 35 |
|---|---|---|---|---|---|---|---|---|---|---|---|---|---|---|---|---|---|
| | | | | | | | | (Overweight)* | | | | (Obese) | | | | | |
| 4'10" (58") | 91 | 96 | 100 | 105 | 110 | 115 | 119 | 124 | 129 | 134 | 138 | **143** | **148** | **153** | **158** | **162** | **167** |
| 4'11" (59") | 94 | 99 | 104 | 109 | 114 | 119 | 124 | 128 | 133 | 138 | 143 | **148** | **153** | **158** | **163** | **168** | **173** |
| 5' (60") | 97 | 102 | 107 | 112 | 118 | 123 | 128 | 133 | 138 | 143 | 148 | **153** | **158** | **163** | **168** | **174** | **179** |
| 5'1" (61") | 100 | 106 | 111 | 116 | 122 | 127 | 132 | 137 | 143 | 148 | 153 | **158** | **164** | **169** | **174** | **180** | **185** |
| 5'2" (62") | 104 | 109 | 115 | 120 | 126 | 131 | 136 | 142 | 147 | 153 | 158 | **164** | **169** | **175** | **180** | **186** | **191** |
| 5'3" (63") | 107 | 113 | 118 | 124 | 130 | 135 | 141 | 146 | 152 | 158 | 163 | **169** | **175** | **180** | **186** | **191** | **197** |
| 5'4" (64") | 110 | 116 | 122 | 128 | 134 | 140 | 145 | 151 | 157 | 163 | 169 | **174** | **180** | **186** | **192** | **197** | **204** |
| 5'5" (65") | 114 | 120 | 126 | 132 | 138 | 144 | 150 | 156 | 162 | 168 | 174 | **180** | **186** | **192** | **198** | **204** | **210** |
| 5'6" (66") | 118 | 124 | 130 | 136 | 142 | 148 | 155 | 161 | 167 | 173 | 179 | **186** | **192** | **198** | **204** | **210** | **216** |
| 5'7" (67") | 121 | 127 | 134 | 140 | 146 | 153 | 159 | 166 | 172 | 178 | 185 | **191** | **198** | **204** | **211** | **217** | **223** |
| 5'8" (68") | 125 | 131 | 138 | 144 | 151 | 158 | 164 | 171 | 177 | 184 | 190 | **197** | **203** | **210** | **216** | **223** | **230** |
| 5'9" (69") | 128 | 135 | 142 | 149 | 155 | 162 | 169 | 176 | 182 | 189 | 196 | **203** | **209** | **216** | **223** | **230** | **236** |
| 5'10" (70") | 132 | 139 | 146 | 153 | 160 | 167 | 174 | 181 | 188 | 195 | 202 | **209** | **216** | **222** | **229** | **236** | **243** |
| 5'11" (71") | 136 | 143 | 150 | 157 | 165 | 172 | 179 | 186 | 193 | 200 | 208 | **215** | **222** | **229** | **236** | **243** | **250** |
| 6' (72") | 140 | 147 | 154 | 162 | 169 | 177 | 184 | 191 | 199 | 206 | 213 | **221** | **228** | **235** | **242** | **250** | **258** |
| 6'1" (73") | 144 | 151 | 159 | 166 | 174 | 182 | 189 | 197 | 204 | 212 | 219 | **227** | **235** | **242** | **250** | **257** | **265** |
| 6'2' (74") | 148 | 155 | 163 | 171 | 179 | 186 | 194 | 202 | 210 | 218 | 225 | **233** | **241** | **249** | **256** | **264** | **272** |
| 6'3' (75") | 152 | 160 | 168 | 176 | 184 | 192 | 200 | 208 | 216 | 224 | 232 | **240** | **248** | **256** | **264** | **272** | **279** |

| BMI | Meaning |
|---|---|
| 19 - 25 | Normal weight |
| 26 - 29 | Overweight |
| 30 + | Obese |

Note the * beside the (Overweight) range of 26-29 BMI. It is important to remember that Body Mass Index has its limitations. Athletes with more muscle mass are going to have a disproportionately higher BMI due to the fact that muscle weighs more than fat. And likewise an elderly or inactive person with decreased muscle mass may have a disproportionately low BMI.

You may wonder, with all its limitations why I consider the BMI as a helpful tool in determining healthy weight range. Simply, the medical and insurance communities continue to use BMI to define healthy weight ranges. Because of this, you need to be familiar with it.

In addition, one advantage that a BMI range has over mere numbers on a weight scale is that it takes into consideration one's height.

For myself, I consistently fall into the "overweight" range on the BMI chart. I do not stress and obsess about it. I spent years at a BMI of 35 and experienced the negative health effects of those extra pounds. Now I use the BMI chart as a point of reference as I continue to strive to live a balanced lifestyle while being mindful of my personal family disease risk factors.

Over time, I have learned to be happy with myself and no longer expend precious energy on the "Size 6 ideal" I used to strive for. It does help that I have *never* been a size 6.

Let your idea of perfection go. Adopt a balanced view of your *own* perfection. What is perfect for you will not exactly match everyone else. So focusing your energy on a number will only trap you in disappointment and blind you from seeing and appreciating the real progress you are making. Be realistic about who you are, where you find yourself right now and what a more balanced weight range might be for you.

## Tool #2: Waist Circumference

An accurate measurement of your waist circumference is another important tool in weight and health risk assessment. Not surprisingly, this is also largely determined by your genetics.

You may have heard that if you body has more of a "pear" shape than an "apple" shape, you will have a greater health advantage. This is true. Abdominal fat – the fat that accumulates around your waist and stomach – increases your risk for diabetes, heart disease, sleep apnea and hormonal disorders which could lead to cancer, even if you are at a healthy weight.

*Generally*, women have more fat distributed in their lower body while men's fat accumulates around their bellies. As women age and their estrogen decreases, however, their bodies may begin to store more fat around their middles.

## Calculate your waist circumference

To measure your waist circumference, place a cloth tape measure around your bare abdomen an inch above your hip bones and relax. The tape should be snug, but not pushing tightly into the skin. Make sure the tape is parallel to the floor. For accuracy, measure three times then take the average. Compare your findings with the guidelines below.

### Dangerous Waist Size

| Women | Men |
|:---:|:---:|
| 35 inches and above | 40 inches and above |

Similar to the Body Mass Index, waist circumference has its limitations, but it is widely accepted as a better indicator of health risks than BMI alone.

## Tool #3: Body Fat Percentage

Another indicator of your health is how much of your body weight is actually fat. Too much body fat increases our weight which in turn leads to increased disease risk. Increasing weight *a little* as you age is fine to a certain extent as long as you stay within a healthy weight range.

Simply put, when you eat and drink more calories than your body needs the excess is stored as body fat. Body fat is once again greatly affected by your genetic makeup. If you lined up a dozen

30 year old men who are 5' 10' and 200 lbs and measured their body fat percentages, you would get 30 different results.

Before you think that fat itself is your great enemy, you need to know that your body needs fat. It is extremely important to bodily functions. That is why, if you notice the chart below, a healthy woman in her forties or fifties may have as much as 23-35% body fat. It is not fat itself, but the proportion of fat in your body that you need to monitor.

## Women

| Age | Healthy Range | Overweight | Obese |
|-----|---------------|------------|-------|
| 20-40 yrs | 21-33% | 33-39% | Over 39% |
| 41-60 yrs | 23-35% | 35-40% | Over 40% |
| 61-79 yrs | 24-36% | 36-42% | Over 42% |

## Men

| Age | Healthy Range | Overweight | Obese |
|-----|---------------|------------|-------|
| 20-40 yrs | 8-19% | 19-25% | Over 25% |
| 41-60 yrs | 11-22% | 22-27% | Over 27% |
| 61-79 yrs | 13-25% | 25-30% | Over 30% |

It is a good idea to monitor your body fat percentage two or three times a year. There are weight scales available at most large stores and from various websites you can use in your own home. They use bioelectrical impedance to determine one's body fat and body water percentage.

Many reputable fitness facilities have professionals who are trained to provide this service. Some local universities or colleges also provide even more accurate calculations of your body fat percentage. Our local university, Appalachian State, offers various testing to the public for a fee, such as underwater weighing.

## What to Do With Your Information

As you can see, relying on what you read on your bathroom scale or even the charts in your doctor's office should not be the only factor when determining a balanced, healthy weight range. All three of these calculations: body mass index, body fat percentage and waist circumference are very helpful for creating a more complete picture of your health risks.

Now that you have collected your personal statistics, what should you do?

- First, *write down* your findings and document how they change as you begin to adopt balanced and healthier lifestyle habits.

- Second, if you haven't had a physical in a while, schedule one and share the information you have gathered with your doctor.

## To Sum Up

Being your own best advocate means accepting responsibility for your health. No one knows your body like you do, so assume your role as the expert of your own body and step out to change the things that you can change.

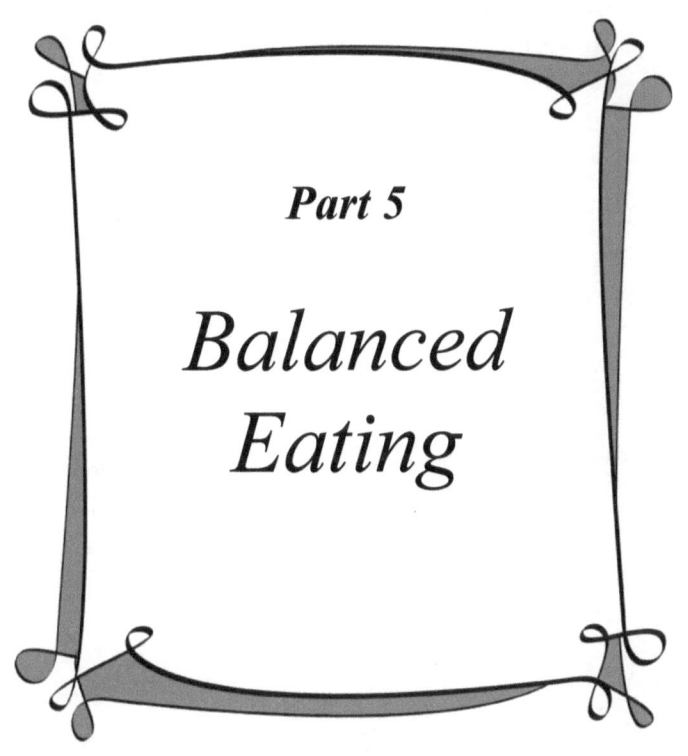

**Part 5**

*Balanced*
*Eating*

# Chapter 12

# For the Love of Food

*"Leave the gun. Take the cannolis."*
*~ Clemenza, in The Godfather*

Imagine it: warm bread from the oven, a freshly sliced tomato, a 4th of July burger straight from the grill, plucking a plump blueberry from the plant and popping it in your mouth, soft and gooey chocolate chip cookies.

Ahh, food – no matter how you slice it (pun intended) food invokes a reaction. Is it any wonder why the first date for many people looking for romance involves sharing a meal together? Why do people bring food to friends when they have lost a loved one? The bride and groom slice the wedding cake and feed it to each other. Name any nationality, ethnic group or culture and their traditions involving food will be part of the description. Food is more than just fuel for our bodies.

Some of my life's most cherished memories continue to be formed while sharing food with family and friends I treasure.

Humans are blessed with the ability to truly savor and enjoy a myriad of foods and drinks. European cultures traditionally take their time while sitting down to share a meal. They enjoy the smells, the mixture of flavors and good conversation. Americans, especially those of us who want to adopt a healthier lifestyle approach to eating, should learn from these other cultures.

Are "fast" and "big" the primary words we want associated with our American relationship with food? As we have spread our fast food around the globe obesity, cancer and heart disease have increased as well.

As a wellness professional I regularly feel torn between my own passion for foods, the honest joy of preparing and sharing foods with others and my responsibility to promote what I know are sound eating habits.

This inspired my title choice, "I Want to Have My Cake & Lose Weight Too." With time and experience I have happily discovered that food and all its joys can coexist with a commitment to lose weight. The key is balance.

This is no small challenge in a media environment that promotes extremes. On one hand we hear, "Eat as much as you want," "No need to exercise," "Just pop this pill," "Just sprinkle this on." While at the same time other popular diets proclaim, "Remove this food or list of foods entirely from your diet," "Eat no more than 500 calories per day while you take this supplement," "You must perform this exercise daily for 90 minutes." It is no wonder people don't know what to believe. Where is the balance?

## "Good" and "Bad" Food

Health promotion professionals often make a choice to promote that various foods and drinks are either *good or bad.* The trouble with this all-or-nothing approach is that it implies that *you* must be bad if you choose something from the *bad* group of foods. Consider the relationship with food a child develops as they witness this viewpoint expressed on a daily basis.

I often feel like a priest in a confessional when someone takes my arm and pulls me aside to whisper, "I've been bad." The person then rattles off all the food and drink sins they have committed in an attempt to unburden themselves of their guilt by confessing to me. I am often tempted, in the spirit of the moment, to reply, "For your penance, eat one cup of carrots, drink 4 glasses of water and have no desserts for a week!" But instead I try to encourage them to let go of their guilt and move forward with the understanding that looking at food as *good or bad* is definitely not balanced or healthy.

Some in our field feel strongly that the human race is incapable of striking a proper balance, so the only solution is for us to eliminate all "unhealthy" foods and drinks.

As an eternal optimist I wholeheartedly believe that we can learn to have balance as we make the daily, real-life choices concerning what we put in our mouths.

I feel just as strongly that finding that balance must be determined on an individual basis. If you are aware of a strong family history of disease, like diabetes, or if you have been informed of a medical condition that is directly related to your lifestyle choices, it is even more important to make consistent, healthy choices.

Now we come to the million dollar question – How can we possibly balance the foods and beverages we eat, the various nutrients our bodies need to survive and thrive, while satisfying our undeniable joy of eating?

## Look at the Big Picture

The balanced approach is choosing to make healthy, daily choices the majority of the time. A healthy lifestyle looks at the big picture.

Believe me, if the criteria for wellness and lifestyle coaching required daily perfection in our eating there would be no professionals in the wellness field. No one is perfect. I don't make what some would consider, "perfectly healthy" food and drink choices every minute of every day. But I do focus on a healthy lifestyle, am honest with myself and the purposeful choices I make while keeping my self-talk positive.

With balance you can evaluate your week as a whole. There is no need to beat yourself up over a choice or two. I cannot stress enough how important it is to give yourself a break. Allow yourself to enjoy a nice meal at a restaurant with your family and friends. Savor the piece of cake you share with an old friend when you meet for lunch. And, if you make a purposeful decision to grab the junk food impulse buy at the counter while you're paying for your gas, own it and move on.

Guilt and shame are not part of a healthy, balanced lifestyle. If you find yourself making some consistently unhealthy choices for a few days, reevaluate and choose to begin making small changes that will get you back on track tomorrow. Recognize the distinct difference between eating out of habit or because the food is simply there and making purposeful decisions as part of a healthier lifestyle. There is no magic formula; you have to make the choice.

## Why Are You Eating?

I have asked *many* people who have never had an issue with their weight why they don't overeat. Their typical response goes something like this: "I eat when I'm hungry and I really don't think about it." This response is quite different from many people who are overweight who tell me that they eat for eating's sake.

Perhaps emotions are involved, perhaps stress, but most of the time it is simply because the food is present. Many clients have told me that even as they are eating, they are thinking about their next meal. In a generally wealthy culture like the United States, food is abundant and available. It has become an end in itself. We have essentially forgotten what it feels like, physically, to be hungry.

I would wager that most of us eat both because we're hungry and out of habit. Maybe your daily routine includes stopping for a high-calorie latte on the way to work, a high-fat dessert with your coffee every night or you indulge a craving to try to cope with some emotional void or problem. Maybe the soft drink you occasionally drank at the office has now become a staple on your desk or you and your coworkers eat out daily for lunch. Maybe you have never left food on your plate or the rest of your drink in your glass because you've been reared to consider it wasteful.

Whatever your choices may be, the majority of us do not eat just because we are hungry.

Here are some guidelines to assist you in an honest evaluation of your choices. Use the lists below to help you determine when and why you are eating.

### Signs of Physical Hunger

1. Grows gradually, hours after a meal
2. Feel it in your growling stomach or low energy level
3. Is not based on habit
4. Goes away when you feel satisfied or full

## Signs of Unhealthy Emotional or Habitual Hunger
1. Develops suddenly
2. Based on your feelings and has nothing to do with physical hunger
3. Has nothing to do with the length of time since you last ate
4. Often accompanied by a craving for a specific food
5. Continues even when full or satisfied
6. Leads to feelings of guilt, shame and embarrassment

Does this mean you should never eat if you're not in actual need of energy? No! I want to clarify that balanced eating allows for eating when you may not be physically hungry. Did I just hear a gasp?! Come on, how many of us have enjoyed a delicious dessert even though we weren't actually hungry? The imbalance is when we choose two or three servings of that delicious dessert or perpetuate habits which lead to certain weight gain, health problems and increased disease risk.

Our balanced, overall goal should be to learn to identify the difference between physical and emotional hunger and develop awareness of why we are actually eating.

Much of our eating, especially in American culture, is simply due to the fact that we are surrounded by ready-to-be-consumed, packaged foods. With balance we begin to focus on what our body needs to survive and thrive and practice portion control.

# Arriving at Moderation

Years ago I led a weight management program at the largest YMCA in the country at the time, the Harris Y in Charlotte, NC.

I remember one of the participants, Alice. I constantly encouraged Alice to give up the diet mentality. She had yo-yo dieted for decades, sliding between eating whatever was in front of her and depriving herself while dieting. Alice had never experienced a truly balanced view of eating in her adult life. During our group sessions she would often raise her hand, interrupt and ask, "Don't you mean that we should *avoid* that food?" I would say, "No, just remember to use portion control." She would look at me suspiciously as if she were mentally scrolling through my list of credentials, wondering if I was qualified to teach a weight management class.

At the end of one meeting she approached me and said, "You will be so proud of me, Gretchen. I'm going to a wedding this weekend and I am not going to allow myself to eat *anything* at the wedding."

After gathering my thoughts, I replied, "Alice, you've dieted and dieted most of your adult life and it is time you stopped depriving yourself. Weddings have some of the best spread there is! Eat mindfully during the day, save up some of those calories to enjoy the food at the wedding, maybe even a small piece of wedding cake and enjoy your time with your friends."

Her eyes grew huge! She was in shock that I, the person who was supposed to be helping her succeed on her *DIET*, was encouraging her to eat – and at a wedding of all places! I continued smiling and nodding and she left with her jaw still dropped. I knew she would have to process my advice and would hopefully gain insight into *why* she struggled between the all or none diet mentality.

The next week Alice came to the group meeting, weighed in and had lost another pound. I kept my eyes down at the clipboard as I recorded her weight and asked, "How was the wedding?" She replied with a deep breath, "I had a great time, and I ate the food in moderation, and I even allowed myself a little piece of cake." She was almost in tears. Alice had a breakthrough. She had finally started her journey, after dieting for most of her adult life, to a realistic approach to weight management.

## To Sum Up

The enjoyment of food is natural. Develop a healthier relationship with food as you honestly examine *why* you are eating. Look at the big picture as you accept responsibility for your balanced choices. Make "moderation" a key word as you move forward on your journey.

**Chapter 13**

# Actually Having *and Enjoying* Your Cake

*Life is too short to pass on a really great dessert.*
*Enjoy it, savor it, share it with someone you love.*

Years ago I purchased my children's birthday cakes from a small bakery. They made the most amazing cakes you have ever tasted – filled with all kinds of deliciousness and the thickest butter cream icing known to man. I'm not kidding – the icing on their cupcakes was as tall as the actual cupcake! Needless to say, it tasted *really* good – drooling good. As you can imagine, a cake that good costs *much* more than your average local, grocery store bakery cake. A cake that decadent and pricey is reserved for special occasions.

This is how we must think when choosing high-calorie, high-fat, high-salt or high-sugar foods and drinks in our daily lives. We can enjoy them in moderation and not feel guilty, but in balance; *not* every day or even every week.

## Individually Determined Moderation

Anyone who has ever allowed me to share my passion about weight management has heard me say: "Any food or drink is fine in moderation." I truly believe this. BUT, and here is the big BUT, I always clarify that each person must be fully aware of their own health status and genetic makeup in order to make the best choices for themselves.

I also clarify that one person's definition of moderation will clearly differ from another's. One person may define moderate eating as choosing to have dessert only once a week while another may define it as having dessert after dinner every day.

Initially it may sound like the first definition is the better choice. But what if that one dessert per week is a half gallon of decadent, high-fat, creamy ice cream topped with hot fudge, while the other's daily serving of dessert is a small piece of organic, dark chocolate to satisfy their sweet tooth? Do you see what I mean? There are many factors to take into consideration as we discuss moderation.

## The Binge

Binge eating is a sensitive subject, but one I feel I must discuss briefly. There are many, many individuals who eat excessive amounts of food from time to time, binging only once in a while, and attempt to justify it by claiming, "all things are fine in moderation."

This is different from food addiction because these people who justify an occasional binge don't feel shame about it. But I must give you the tough truth that there is no place in a healthy lifestyle for binge eating. I know this is hitting a nerve with some of you – it should.

Do not deceive yourself. Consuming large amounts of unhealthy food is *not* okay. I challenge you to be honest with yourself and consider if you have justified your binge eating by cramming it into *your* definition of moderation.

# The Behavior Chain Tool

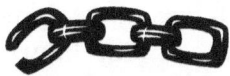

One of the most valuable tools to help you balance and modify your behavior is to understand the chain of events which led to your not-so-healthy choices or habits.

Dr. Kelly Brownell, respected weight management expert, developed this learning tool. It allows you to pin-point, by working *backwards* through a sequence of events, choices, circumstances and behaviors, where the issue began. I have often used this exercise in my work with individuals and small groups.

I'll use myself as an example. One of my habits that causes me frustration is the tendency to make an impulse buy at a gas station convenience store or off the grocery store check-out line shelf. The food disappears so quickly that I don't have time to enjoy it. Even worse, I hardly remember scarfing it down.

If I take the time to fill in my behavior chain it looks something like this:

- Final Link in the Chain
  Upset that I ate something incredibly unhealthy and I didn't even enjoy it

- Previous Link
  Justified stopping for gas or groceries

- Previous Link
  I was hungry

- Previous Link
  I was rushing home from work

- Previous Link
  It was a busy day and I skipped lunch
  Do you see the "ah-ha" moment?

There have been numerous times when I have skipped breakfast or lunch due to a busy schedule or poor time management. We've all been there. I know that when I skip a meal I am going to be hungry. It almost always leads to an impulse buy later. Knowing this about myself and how I end up feeling at the end of this sequence of events prompts me to plan a little better the next time.

Use the behavior chain to pinpoint your habitual not-so-healthy behaviors. I promise it will help you along your path to self-discovery. It will serve to shine a light on some areas you have been eager to identify and change.

## Oh, Well – Now You've Gone from Preachin' to Meddlin'

Jan wanted my assistance to help her lose 10 or 15 pounds to get into a healthier weight range. Her weight loss goal was realistic and balanced and she had completed a recent, thorough physical. She had reduced her caloric intake moderately, was exercising consistently and had even changed up her routine a little, but for some reason she had hit a plateau.

Over the initial first weeks we reviewed her weekly food diaries, examined her exercise routine, discussed techniques to handle the stress on her job, reviewed her sleep habits and even discussed her personal relationships to try to uncover any hidden sabotaging factors. I was at a loss. Why wasn't she losing weight?

Finally, after a little bit of grilling during one of our sessions, she finally revealed an interesting tid-bit she had tried very hard to hide. Every single morning Jan ritualistically drove to her local convenience store and purchased a 64 oz. soda. She had been doing this literally for years and years and did not want to let it go.

Jan concealed this habitual sugar consumption from me until I finally pried it out of her.

Why did she hide it, even though she knew it was sabotaging her weight-loss efforts? Because she didn't want to give it up. It was something she enjoyed – something that was a ritual in her day – a habit – something that made her *feel good*.

It also served as a serious upper of sugar and caffeine. You don't have to be a nutritionist to calculate that a 64 oz. soda equates to a whopping 800+ calories per day.

My advice to Jan – find the balance. No one is saying that you have to go without soft drinks for the rest of your life, but the daily intake of that many calories would have definitely made it difficult to reach a healthier weight. Also, Jan had to be honest with herself about the very serious health consequences from pouring mounds of sugar and caffeine through her system daily.

It was time – time for Jan to gradually wean herself from the soda she had become addicted to and practice moderation.

Oh, it was painful. During one of our subsequent sessions together Jan informed me that she had gone through so much psychological and physical withdrawal that she fashioned a small voodoo doll replica of me to torture. I responded unnervingly, "Hey, whatever it takes!"

When Jan started reducing the amount of soft drinks, which reduced her daily calories, she began to gradually lose weight even with no additional changes in her lifestyle.

## Make *New* Habits

Remember that it takes time to establish new habits as you continue on your journey to a healthier lifestyle.

Jan had to learn to replace an unbalanced, unhealthy habit with a healthier alternative. She had to replace her habitual soft drink consumption with something else. This is a common predicament for many people who discover many of their additional calories are coming from what they are drinking, whether it is the specialty coffee they pick up every morning on their way to work, the creamer they add to their coffee at home, the large glass of wine with dinner, the beer or two with friends after work or the daily soft drink or sweet tea with their meals.

When someone asks for my alternative I always have the same answer – drink water. I don't care what it takes – learn to develop the habit of giving your body six to eight cups of healthy water a day. Establish this daily habit *first* and then make purposeful decisions when choosing an additional beverage through your day.

The same applies to food choices. Break your daily sugar and salt habits by replacing them with healthier alternatives. Make sure you are getting in a couple pieces of fruit per day and a few servings of vegetables. I know fruits and veggies don't seem as appealing as the bag of chips from the vending machine, the candy bar from the check-out line at the grocery store or the fries from the drive-thru (and no, french fries and ketchup do not count as two vegetable servings). Stick with it and you will begin to feel so much better.

Make the choice to improve your health by adopting healthy water, fruits and vegetables as a foundation for your daily, healthy habits. After these are part of your typical day you will find your ability to make more purposeful choices will improve.

## To Sum Up

Continue to accept responsibility for your choices. Habits can be hard to change, especially when they've been a part of your daily life for a long time, but you can do it. Have patience and don't give up as you replace your old habits with healthier alternatives.

# Chapter 14

# Grocery Shopping
# The Entry Versus the Exit

*"The odds of going to the store for a loaf of bread and
coming out with only a loaf of bread
are three billion to one."*
~ Erma Bombeck

There is a reason I am placing this chapter on grocery shopping in the section on *Balanced Eating* and not *Balanced Nutrition*. Mrs. Bombeck could not have put it better: What are the chances of us actually coming out of that temptation filled building with only one item? Slim to none. On those few occasions I have actually achieved this feat, I have celebrated in the parking lot with a loud "YESSS!"

Grocery shopping is not for the weak. It is not for the unprepared. What you purchase in your local grocery store is what you will have around the house and reach for when you are hungry, bored or attempting to comfort yourself emotionally.

But do not fear – you are not alone. Grocery shopping is something the majority of us do so poorly that it is no wonder we struggle to maintain a healthy weight.

The ability to purposefully navigate through the grocery store minefield will serve as a powerful tool as you move forward with healthier habits.

Have you ever watched one of those intervention shows where the registered dietician or nutritionist come in to a family's home and begins to place all the "not-so-healthy" foods in black garbage bags? I know; it is hard for me to watch too, especially when the family's food supply goes from stocked shelves in the refrigerator and pantry to a bottle of water on the door of the fridge, an ice tray in the freezer and one, lonely can of tuna on the pantry shelf. It can be brutal.

Why is it important to begin by removing those foods from the family's home? Because our homes *should be* the one place where we are eating most of our meals and snacks so our food choices need to be, for the most part, easier.

Use the following tips to make sure you are filling your home with foods that are healthy for your body and spirit.

## Grocery Shopping 101

1. Try to Plan Your Week
   This is probably the most important part of grocery shopping. Do it before you leave the house. You know what you like to eat. Eating and cooking at home will help you manage your weight. Take the time to plan the meals you are going to prepare for the week, or at least the basic ingredients for a few main meals you will enjoy so you won't feel tempted to grab high-calorie, prepackaged items. Remember: shop with purpose.

2. Do not go hungry
   You will make poor food-buying choices when you head into the grocery store with no list, no plan and no food in your belly.

3. Make a list
   Now that you have an idea of your meals and snacks for the week, prepare your store list. *Write it down.* Try to purchase as much organic food as you can afford. Your weekly list should contain these basics:

   • Fresh fruits – Check to see which fruits are in season as they will be a lot cheaper. For instance, berries are wonderful for your health and are least expensive in the summer.

- Fresh vegetables
  If you can afford it, purchase some veggies that are already bite-size like baby carrots, broccoli and cauliflower. You will be more likely to eat them if you don't have to do the prep work. The same goes for the prepared bags of leaf lettuce. Do not hide them in the hydrator drawer; place them on the top shelf to grab as a quick snack. Some great news – almost all grocery stores are carrying organically grown, ready-to-eat vegetables.

- Whole grains
  Contrary to popular belief, carbohydrates are not evil. Keep a loaf of whole grain bread on hand. Cereal made with whole grains is another good staple. These items are quick and easy to prepare.

- Dairy products
  Choose reduced and low fat milks, cheeses and yogurts. Two percent milk is not low fat, but it is reduced fat, which makes it a better choice than whole milk. Read the labels on yogurts as many of them have artificial sweeteners which should be avoided.

- Beverages
  Avoid bringing soft drinks into your home and avoid diet sodas all together – they are not a healthier choice. If you are going to select a fruit juice, choose one that is 100% juice with no added sugars.

- Proteins
  Eggs are a great source of protein. Choose chicken, fish and lean cuts of beef. Purchase only rarely processed meats like luncheon meat, hotdogs, bacon and sausages.

- Frozen foods
  Stock up on frozen vegetables. Buy poultry and lean meats when they are on sale and store them in your freezer.

- Oils
  Always keep a jar of olive oil in your pantry for cooking. Read the food labels on salad dressings and choose ones with healthful ingredients, rather than those that contain cheap hydrogenated oils and sugars.

- Snack items
  Nuts, seeds, fresh fruits and vegetables are your best bet to have on-hand. If you like an occasional cracker, there are healthier, baked options available. Just read your ingredient list and avoid partially hydrogenated oils and added salt and sugars.

- Jars and Cans
  These are very convenient. Some of the new organic red pasta sauces even rival my home-made sauce! Cans of tuna packed in water and salt-free or reduced sodium vegetables and soups are great staples for your pantry shelf.

4. Avoid the landmines
   If you haven't noticed, the middle aisle of your grocery store is commonly the chip and soda aisle. Producers of these products are hoping that you will walk down this middle aisle on your way to some

other part of the store and will succumb to the impulse buy. Also, notice the placement of the brightly colored, sugar-packed, kid's cereals. They are purposely placed on shelves at a child's eye level to entice kids to grab a box. Take your kids and grandkids to the store with you and teach them how to make healthy, balanced choices.

5.  Do not be fooled by the marketing
    "Smart" and "enhanced." Do these claims actually mean anything or is it simply clever marketing? No one regulates these claims so be careful not to fall for the flashy writing on the front of the package. Read your label. Determine what is actually inside the product you are purchasing. The term "natural" does have to meet criteria regarding artificial or synthetic ingredients (including all color additives regardless of their source). But just because something is labeled *natural* does not mean it may be the healthiest choice.

## Know Your Food Labels

If you have not learned how to read the food labels at the grocery store, now is the time.

Food marketing professionals work hard to catch your eye as you walk down the aisles of your grocery store. Their main purpose, of course, is to entice you to buy whatever product they are selling. Do not trust what you read on the front packaging of every box, bag, jar or can you pass. Take the time to educate yourself about food labels so you are equipped to make wiser and healthier choices.

The United States Food and Drug Administration (FDA) requires most packaged food and beverage items to have the "Nutrition Facts" label.

Food label guidelines have toughened over the years and will continue to change as advocacy groups pressure for stricter labeling. This is a good thing because as long as money is involved there will be attempts to deliberately deceive the public with creative advertising tactics.

One of the best examples of deceptive advertising was the "no cholesterol" marketing that sky rocketed in the 1990's. The dangers of high cholesterol became a popular media message due to a combination of consumer health advocacy and advertising. Suddenly food manufacturers found ways to label many foods *cholesterol free* as a way to cash in on public anxiety about cholesterol.

Even products made of fruits, vegetables and grains that never had any cholesterol in them were labeled this way. Some manufacturers even promoted products as *cholesterol free* that contained trans fats. Sadly, we knew twenty years ago that trans fats were known to raise LDL or "bad" cholesterol, and reduce HDL or "good" cholesterol. Manufacturers implied through their labeling that their food, by being "cholesterol free" was more healthful than other foods. Nothing could have been less true.

The ever continuing butter versus margarine debate is another prime example. Food manufacturers promoted margarine as a healthier alternative to butter because it did not contain saturated fat and cholesterol. But the truth about margarine was and still is that it does contain trans fats which, as stated, increases "bad" cholesterol when you eat it and reduces your "good" cholesterol.

Those of us in the health promotion field have long been aware of the need for stricter labeling, and we celebrate the fact that now trans fats are listed with saturated fat and cholesterol on the nutrition facts panel.

However, labels will only help consumers if they know how to accurately interpret them.

Familiarize yourself with the following Nutrition Facts Panel. Start at the top of this snack label and work your way down.

**Nutrition Facts**

Serving Size 1 ounce   Servings in bag 4

**Amount Per Serving**

| | | |
|---|---|---|
| **Calories 155** | Calories from Fat 93 | |
| | | **% Daily Value*** |
| **Total Fat** 11g | | 16% |
| Saturated Fat 3g | | 15% |
| Trans Fat | | |
| **Cholesterol** 0mg | | 0% |
| **Sodium** 148mg | | 6% |
| **Total Carbohydrate** 14g | | 5% |
| Dietary Fiber 1g | | 5% |
| Sugars 1g | | |
| **Protein** 2g | | |

| | | | |
|---|---|---|---|
| Vitamin A | 0% | • Vitamin C | 9% |
| Calcium | 1% | • Iron | 3% |

* Percent Daily Values are based on a 2,000 calorie diet. Your daily values may be higher or lower depending on your calorie needs.

- Serving Size
  This is one of the most important parts of the food label that people skip right over. This bag contains four servings of this snack item. If you eat the entire bag you need to multiply all the other nutrition facts by four.

- Calories
  One serving contains 155 calories. If you ate the entire bag your total caloric intake from this snack is 620 calories – about one third of your reduced calorie daily goal for a woman.

- Fat
  If you stopped at one serving you would have consumed 11 grams of fat, but if you ate the whole bag that is a whopping 44 grams of fat, 12 of which are artery-clogging saturated fat grams. That is more fat than you should eat in your whole day.

Taking the time to skim over the current nutrition panel is helpful, especially when focusing on portion and serving sizes. Thankfully the food labels will continue to be revised in an attempt to make them as user-friendly as possible.

## The Ingredients List – What are You *Really* Eating?

You have scanned the food nutrition panel and think you have figured out what is going on inside that little box, can, jar or wrapper you hold in your hand.

Now it is time to take it one step further and read the ingredients list. It may be the most important clue you need in order to make an informed choice about this food or drink before you put it in your body.

Many are surprised to learn that the ingredients are listed in order of weight from greatest to least. If sugar is listed as the first ingredient, then there is more sugar, by weight, than any other ingredient in that product. Some advertisers will promote the addition of a healthful ingredient, but upon careful examination of the ingredient list may find it listed *last*. Meaning it doesn't contain much of it at all.

## Are You Getting Too Much of These?

We Americans love to eat our sugar, salt and fat, but have a difficult time finding a balance. Realize that too much will make you overweight and contribute to other health problems.

There is certainly a place for the occasional decadent item in a balanced, real-life approach to weight management. Just remember the key term is "occasional."

The American Heart Association (AHA) has provided suggested limits for the following ingredients. If you cannot remember these helpful guidelines *write each one down* on a piece of paper and put it in your wallet or purse. Keep it handy so you can review it during your next trip to the store. It will not take long to learn these guidelines so that you will no longer need to refer to your list.

## Added Sugar

- Women – No more than 24 grams of sugar
  (about 6 teaspoons or 100 calories per day)
- Men – No more than 36 grams of sugar
  (about 9 teaspoons or 150 calories per day)

Sugar has a place in a balanced, healthy lifestyle, but not in excess. Your body and brain needs sugar to function, but it gets what it needs from the variety of foods you eat. Most of us eat way too much added sugar. The more you eat, the more you want and will crave it.

Excess sugar can lead to hormonal imbalances, depression, high blood pressure and even an increase in arterial damage. Add to that the empty calories that your body stores as extra weight and you begin to see that practicing moderation is a must when it comes to sugar.

Sure, we all know those foods that contain large amounts of sugar like sodas, cereals, fruit juices, jellies, canned fruit, cookies, candy, cakes, pies and pastries. But did you know that some of the biggest sugar culprits today are large specialty coffees and the popular, so-called "energy" drinks? You see some of these drinks promoted by athletes or during a sports event on TV, but few of us can claim any benefit from these sugar packed beverages because we aren't professional athletes or marathon runners. Without high levels of activity, the body has no use for all these extra calories and stores them as fat. Even many of the water beverages, which are often marketed as a healthy option because they have added vitamins, are packed with added sugars.

If you are wondering how the soda you had with lunch measures up, one 12 ounce can has more than 9 teaspoons of sugar – three more than your total day's balanced limit. Surprising, isn't it? Add that to the naturally occurring sugars you have consumed in your milk, fruit and other foods which give your body nutrients it can use and needs. The calories from the soda are only adding to your waistline, not giving your body the fuel it craves. Drink soda in extreme moderation and remember to think of each serving as a liquid dessert.

Here are a handful of the most common terms used to disguise sugar in the ingredient list:

| | |
|---|---|
| barley malt | high-fructose corn syrup |
| corn syrup | maltodextrin |
| dextrose | maltose |
| fruit juice concentrate | molasses |
| glucose | sucrose |

A few years ago it was estimated that $229 million dollars were being spent annually marketing sugary cereals to kids. As an example, notice the three ways sugars are listed in one of the most popular breakfast cereals marketed to kids…

Ingredients: MILLED CORN, *SUGAR*, *MALT FLAVORING*, *HIGH FRUCTOSE CORN SYRUP*, SALT, etc.

Sugar, malt flavoring and high fructose corn syrup are three of the top four ingredients by weight. Sure this cereal tastes *grrreat*, but is it a good breakfast choice for kids *or* adults? 12 grams of sugar in just a ¾ cup serving (and who is going to eat only ¾ of a cup), equals 3 teaspoons of sugar in one, small bowl.

As you begin to read your ingredient lists you will discover that sugar is added to practically everything. Manufacturers may try to justify the addition claiming that it preserves freshness or balances flavor, but it all adds up to extra calories. Cutting back on added sugar will help you reduce your weight and make you feel so much better.

An easy tip to remember when determining if the product you are choosing has too much sugar is to use the numbers 15 and 5. If a serving has 15 grams or more of sugar that is high, less than 5 grams is a better choice. Become aware of how much sugar you are honestly consuming in your day.

## Saturated Fat

Not all fats are created equal. Saturated fats can increase your risk for heart disease and Type 2 diabetes. They are found in animal products like egg yolks, beef, pork and high-fat dairy products such as butter and cheese. Some plants like coconut and palm oils also contain saturated fats and are typically found in processed baked goods. Here is your guideline:

- No more than 7% of your daily caloric intake

Most of us in the health promotion field recommend even less than this. Strive for no more than 10 grams of saturated fat per day.

A 3.5 ounce regular hamburger from one of the major fast food chains doesn't stack up too badly at 7 grams of total fat, 3 grams of which are saturated. But choosing the large double patty with cheese gives you 48 grams of fat, 20 grams of which come from artery-clogging saturated fat.

## Cholesterol

Cholesterol assists with the production of hormones and cell membrane functioning. Your body needs cholesterol, but it makes all it needs.

Cholesterol itself is not a fat, but it enters the body from the saturated fatty foods listed above. If something is high in saturated fat it is likely high in cholesterol. When you eat more red meat, shell-fish and butter you increase your risk for heart disease and stroke. The breakfast biscuit you may have picked up at the drive thru this morning on the way to work packs in 555 milligrams of cholesterol. Compare this to your suggested daily intake:

- Less than 300 milligrams per day

- Less than 200 milligrams per day if you are at increased risk for heart disease due to genetic or other risk factors.

Eggs have received a lot of negative press over the amount of cholesterol they contain, but they are an excellent source of protein. All the cholesterol, 210 milligrams, is contained in the yolk of the egg. The good news is that the lecithin contained in the egg prevents the body from absorbing all the cholesterol so one egg a day is a balanced choice for most individuals.

Working in the cardiac rehabilitation field helped me understand the strong genetic component some have with elevated cholesterol. If you already have high cholesterol, or you know you have a strong family history of high cholesterol, be diligent and aware of how much additional cholesterol you are consuming.

## Sodium

Your body needs sodium and regulates the amount it needs, but just like with sugar and fat, we Americans eat way too much salt. Eating too much may lead to high blood pressure and the risk of heart disease and stroke. Even when you avoid adding salt to your food at the table, many of the prepackaged products and canned goods you buy are extremely high in sodium. Restaurants also add a lot of salt to your food before it is ever presented at the table. Your sodium guidelines:

- Less than 2,300 milligrams per day

- Less than 1,500 milligrams per day if you are 51 or over or have high blood pressure

Table salt is probably the biggest source of excess sodium in our American diet. One teaspoon of salt has 2,325 milligrams of sodium. Remove the salt shaker from the table and check the sodium amounts in the sauces, salad dressings, soups and snack foods you purchase to avoid getting too much.

## Avoid Food Additives

*"We are living in a world today where lemonade is made from artificial flavors and furniture polish is made from real lemons."*
*~ Alfred E. Newman, Fictional Cartoon Character,*
*Mad Magazine*

Let's face it, how many of us are able to eat the majority of our food straight from the farm? My bet would be not too many of us, unless you live on the farm or buy all your food at the local farmer's market.

The following is a list of food additives you may find in your ingredients lists and why you should avoid them.

- Sodium nitrite or sodium nitrate
  This is a chemical compound used as a preservative, color and flavor enhancer in the processing of luncheon meats, hot dogs, ham, bacon – basically cured meats and fish in general. This additive may promote cancer cell growth and is becoming an increasing concern.

- Saccharin, Aspartame, Acesulfame-K
  These artificial sweeteners are often referred to as *sugar substitutes*. They are commonly found in "diet" foods, soft drinks, gums, yogurts, etc. The side effects of artificial sweeteners include headaches, migraines and dizziness. Choosing an artificial sweetener is *not* a healthier choice. Many of these sweeteners are hundreds of times sweeter than sugar so our bodies become used to the excessive sweetness and crave more. Instead of using a sugar substitute buy the real thing, in moderation.

- Monosodium Glutamate (MSG)
  MSG is a flavor enhancer commonly found in Chinese food, packaged seasonings, salad dressings, chips, dips, crackers and boxed pasta, hamburger and rice mixes. It actually works by tricking the food receptors in your brain. Side effects range from breathing difficulties, burning sensations, heart palpitations and nausea, to dizziness and overall weakness.

- Caffeine
  Caffeine is a stimulant and occurs naturally in coffee, tea and cocoa. A cup or two of regular coffee a day causes no harm to the body. Some studies have even shown health benefits associated with moderate coffee consumption, due to its antioxidant qualities. Watch out for caffeine that has been added to beverages, like soft drinks. We know caffeine can be mildly addictive, especially when coupled with sugar. Side

effects include restlessness, insomnia, increased heart rate, nausea and vomiting as well as sleep disorders.

- Artificial colors and food dyes
  These synthetic chemicals do not occur in nature and are typically added to junk foods, candy, beverages and baked goods to make them more eye-appealing. You will find them listed as Red 40, Yellow 5, etc. Some individuals, especially children, have shown sensitivities and even extreme allergic reaction to food dyes. Many other countries have banned their use, but the United States still permits them.

## To Sum Up

Educate yourself so you can make better informed choices. Don't trust that the enticing advertising is revealing the whole truth. Read your labels to ensure the items you choose are contributing to your healthy lifestyle.

# Chapter 15

# Eating Out With Balance

*"Dining with one's friends and beloved family*
*is certainly one of life's primal*
*and most innocent delights,*
*one that is both soul-satisfying and eternal."*
~ Julia Child

When you grasp the importance of the big picture in real-life weight management, you begin to enjoy food a little more. The shame, guilt and regret are replaced with positive, honest, moderate choices. You understand the importance of making your body a priority so it can operate at its best. You begin to appreciate that a healthy lifestyle is all about variety and balance.

Eating out is certainly a part of our lives, and rightly so. But it is an area where many give up their control. It doesn't have to be this way. It is not difficult to enjoy yourself at any given restaurant while making overall healthier choices.

Our family did not eat out very often as I was growing up. We were blessed to have the opportunity to sit around the large family table with all seven of us enjoying a family meal together.

Society has changed. We are eating fewer meals at home around the dinner table. More and more of us choose to fill our lives with so many activities and busy work schedules that we have come to *depend* on eating out.

But this has come at a high price. Just as our waistlines have increased in conjunction with increased time sitting at and being entertained by our televisions and computers, the same has occurred with our restaurant habits. Generally speaking, the more you eat out, the more overweight you are likely to be.

The obvious solution is to cook at home and eat at your own table. In doing so, you gain a lot of power over your choices. You know what you're eating and how you prepared it; you can determine your portion sizes much more reasonably; you'll spend a lot less money. In light of the obvious, enjoying a meal out should be viewed as a special occasion.

So how do you eat out in a way that doesn't blow all your best efforts? The key is to be informed and prepared. Restaurant meals usually have more calories, sugar, salt, saturated fat and cholesterol. Also, restaurants rarely give you a choice of fruits, vegetables and low-fat dairy products.

Maybe the most important calorie difference between restaurant meals and home cooked meals is the portion size. It does not matter what restaurant you choose, portion sizes usually far exceed those you would eat at home.

When you understand some of these factors going in to the restaurant, you will be more prepared to make healthier choices and enjoy your restaurant meal much more.

## Gird Your Loins

In other words, *get ready*. Preparation before you go out to eat, especially if you eat out often, is essential when making healthier choices. Some people's careers require them to travel, making eating out a regular necessity. Even if you find yourself in this circumstance you can arm yourself with the same basic guidelines to help you make smarter choices.

The first step is choosing the right place to eat. Avoid restaurants like buffets where your balanced choices are likely to give way to the urge to get your monies worth. Also avoid locations where you know the menu offers very little other than fried options.

Use these easy tips every time you eat out:

- Eat a little less during the day before you eat out
  When I know I am going to enjoy a restaurant dinner I cut back on what I eat during the day, especially at lunch, where I eat only half of what I would normally. I do not recommend skipping meals before eating out because that sets you up to eat much more than you would at the restaurant.

- Be prepared to ask for what you want
  You are the paying customer and most establishments are happy to accommodate reasonable requests. Your restaurant lingo should include the following phrases: "How is that prepared?" "On the side," and "Hold the (fill in the blank)."

- Order some vegetables and/or fruits
  Starting with a salad is usually a good idea depending on the salad. Most restaurants add toppings like bacon, croutons and cheese. Although there is nothing wrong with these in moderation, be prepared to ask for some of the toppings, including the salad dressing, on the side so you can choose how much to use.

- Share the Entree
  The portions offered by most restaurants today provide much more food than any of us should be eating at one sitting. Try sharing the main course. You will easily get a full serving even when you split it.

- Before you start eating, ask for a to-go box
  We all know that if the food is in front of us we will probably eat it, even if we feel satisfied. Ask the server for a to-go container at the same time they bring out your main course and put half of the meal in the box to take home.

## FAST FOOD

> *"You can find your way across this country*
> *using burger joints the way a navigator uses stars."*
> *~ Charles Kuralt*

Ah, those two, simple four-letter words. It is hard to believe there was a time in history when the phrases, *fast food* and *drive-thru* didn't exist yet.

For the most part the fare offered at fast food establishments won't give you the balanced choices you need for a healthy, daily diet. But even fast food can have the occasional place in a balanced lifestyle. When I'm running late to a soccer game with two hungry boys in the car I am glad I have the option of going through the Chic-Fil-A drive-thru.

Thanks in part to public pressure more and more fast food chains offer healthier options on their menus. Kudos to those companies who are going the extra step and posting the nutritional information in plain sight to help us make better choices.

When choosing fast food for your meal use the following information to help you make healthier choices.

## Bigger Portions = Bigger Waistlines

Are you aware of how much fast food portions have changed over the past few decades? Fast food servings are now *three to five times larger* than they were in the 1970's. The average serving size of soda 20 years ago was 6 oz., less than a cup. Today's typical serving is at least 16 oz. Those extra 10 ounces add on around 125 empty calories.

Although I know the fast food industry could be doing more to promote healthier options, there are small strides being made. In particular I am pleased to see smaller items offered on the menus as portion size may be the biggest negative factor of the fast food industry.

- Choose the regular size
  When you "supersize" an item from the fast food menu, the calories, fat, added sugar and salt will be

supersized as well. Avoid doubling the meat and cheeses too, as that greatly increase the amount of saturated fat and cholesterol you will consume.

- Limit the fried sides
  We all enjoy french fries, but enjoying them too often will hurt your health and add to your weight. Balance it out by occasionally choosing a fruit cup, salad or baked potato for a side.

- Choose grilled over fried
  It may surprise you to learn that a hamburger is often lower in fat than a fried chicken or fried fish sandwich. Grilled chicken sandwiches are a much healthier option.

- Skip the mayo and special sauces
  Choose ketchup and mustard instead of high fat condiments.

- Top it with vegetables
  Top your sandwich with lettuce, tomatoes, pickles and onions.

- Ask for the healthier option
  Many more locations are beginning to offer whole grain or whole wheat buns. Choose these instead of the highly processed white breads and buns. Salads, fruit and reduced-fat milk are being offered as healthier alternatives to fries and soda.

## The Drink

So many well-intentioned lifestyle changers forget one important factor when it comes to evaluating the amount of calories they are taking in. They record their foods diligently, they order smaller portions, they ask for high-fat dressings and sauces on the side. In spite of all of their efforts, many neglect to change any of their drink selections. This is especially the case when someone is eating out, whether at a nice restaurant or a fast food chain.

I cannot stress enough the importance of enjoying what you eat and drink in a balanced way when your goal is improved health and weight management.

A soda, one glass of wine – in moderation these are fine. But you have to be honest about how much you allow yourself and your personal definition of "moderate." This applies to those of you who consume alcoholic beverages, but also for those who consume soft drinks, sweetened teas (fellow Southerners please forgive me) and specialty coffees on a regular basis.

Drink calories add up fast! Review the list below to examine where your empty calories are sneaking in:

- Coffee with cream (half-and-half), 12 ounce ~ 40 calories
- Coffee, black, 12 ounce ~ 0-4 calories
- Caffe Latte with whole milk ~ 200 calories
- Energy drink, 12 ounce ~ 160 calories
- Soda, 12 ounce ~ 150 calories
- Bottled sweet tea ~ 135 calories
- Orange Juice, 12 ounce, unsweetened ~ 160 calories
- Whole milk, 12 ounce ~ 220 calories
- 1% milk, 12 ounce ~ 154 calories
- Beer, 12 ounce ~ 153 calories
- Wine, 5 ounce ~ 125 calories

As you can see, the largest amount of liquid recorded in the list above is 12 ounces. Realistically, most sodas today are offered in "convenient" 16 and 20 ounce bottles so choosing convenience will also add additional empty calories. Even 100% juice concentrates the calories and natural fruit sugars are still sugars.

Remember, moderation is the key, even when it comes to your drinks.

## To Sum Up

A healthy lifestyle easily accommodates an occasional meal out. Be aware of the portion sizes you choose from the fast food menu and those served by your waiter or waitress. Prepare during the day by saving up a few calories and enjoy yourself. Be mindful as you choose your beverages and be aware of how many calories you are drinking.

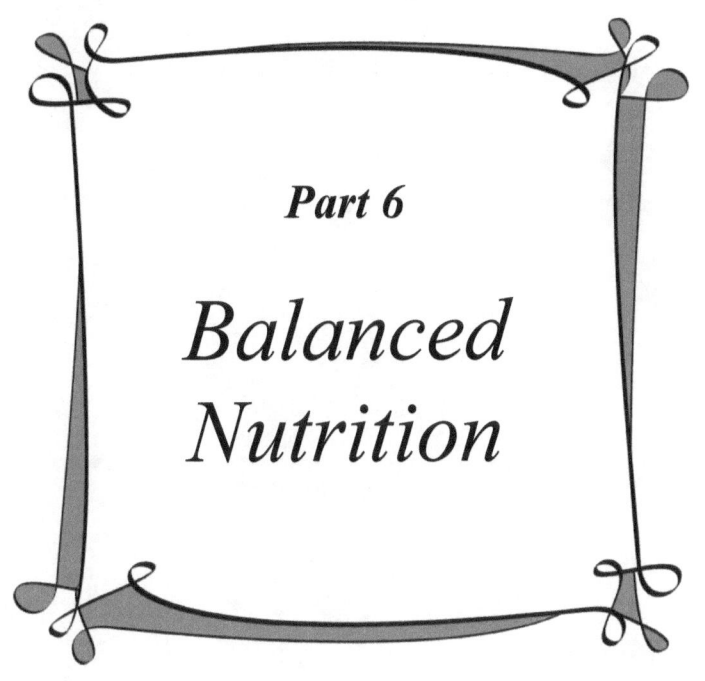

*Part 6*

# *Balanced Nutrition*

# Chapter 16

# Nutrition Basics

*"Don't dig your grave with your own knife and fork."*
*~ English Proverb*

Your physical body is an amazing creation.

To be honest we all abuse and mistreat our bodies to a certain extent instead of giving them the loving care they need to function at their best. When you consider that a small glitch in one of your tiny, intricate cells can wreak havoc on your entire system, you see how much respect your body deserves. Do not wait for your body to break down before taking better care of it.

I like to use the analogy of a car running on fuel. We know that cars can run on more than one type of fuel source; gasoline, ethanol, biofuels, etc. Although it can run on all of these, it processes some faster than others and produces different emissions depending on the fuel source. In an emergency we could even use kerosene or vodka as a temporary fuel source.

Our bodies may be immensely more complex than a car engine, but they operate in a similar manner. We know that our bodies use some fuels more effectively than others. And yet unlike the way in which we care for our cars, we will pour any kind of fuel into our bodies, then trust that our body will take what it needs and filter out the rest.

Yet how many of us would shove a doughnut into the gas tank of our car? Of course your car cannot use any part of a doughnut. So what about your body?

Let's look at what your body does with a doughnut. First, your body receives the doughnut and breaks it down through digestion. It could use the carbohydrates for energy, possibly producing quite a high from the processed sugar. It may use some of the fat for energy as well and then store the excess as body fat.

So yes, your body *can* use a doughnut as fuel the way a car can use kerosene as fuel in an emergency – for a while. But eventually junk food will take a toll on your health.

Unlike a car, your body will store the extra calories you put into it. When you can't get your pants buttoned or you have to slide the belt loop over one more notch toward the end, it should be obvious that you are putting more fuel into your body than it needs or are loading your system with damaging types of fuel.

Besides your weight, think about what is happening under your hood. What about your heart? Just because you cannot see or feel what is slowly building up inside your arteries does not mean it is not happening. Begin to concentrate on what fuel your body needs to operate and function at its best – inside and out.

## Balancing the Basics

One of the biggest mistakes people make when they start focusing on healthier eating is to revert back to a diet mentality. They begin purchasing pounds of lettuce and celery sticks and mentally prepare to deprive themselves of enjoyable foods. But really – who can live on the restrictive guidelines of most diets? That is not balanced. A real-life approach to managing weight entails making healthy choices overall, not living in the shadow of constant deprivation.

I encourage every person I work with to begin their journey toward life-changing balance by *adding* instead of taking away. Do not initially make any other changes.

Begin by *adding* healthy water, fruits and vegetables every day. Very few of us give our bodies enough of these. As you incorporate a variety of foods to fuel your body you will feel better.

## Carbohydrates

*4 Calories per Gram*
*50-60% of Your Daily Calories*

Contrary to what you may have heard over the past decade, carbohydrates are good for you. They are essential to proper bodily functioning, especially for the brain and nervous system. They provide the most available and important source of energy.

Each gram of carbohydrate you eat provides your body with four calories. Carbohydrates should compose about fifty to sixty percent of your daily intake of calories.

But if carbohydrates are so wonderful, why have they received such a bad reputation? You might guess the answer: Because our typical diet doesn't consume them in balance. As with every other choice, balance your carbohydrate intake and learn which sources will do your body the most good.

Carbohydrates can be classified into two main categories:

- Simple Carbohydrates
  Fruits (fructose), vegetables, milk and milk products (lactose) naturally contain this simplest form of carbohydrate. Table sugar (sucrose) is added to foods. Your body uses these sources of carbohydrates rather quickly so you may have heard these carbohydrates called "fast."

- Complex Carbohydrates
  These "slow" carbs provide vitamins, minerals and fiber and produce longer, sustained energy. Unprocessed whole grains, pasta, cereals, vegetables, potatoes, corn and cooked dry beans and peas are great sources of complex carbohydrates.

Nutrition specialists continue to encourage us to eat more *whole grains*, but many people do not know what whole grains are.

Whole grain means exactly what it sounds like: The inside and the outside of the entire grain is used (endosperm, germ and bran) providing vitamins, minerals and fiber – the whole package. A few servings a day of these types of grains have been shown to reduce the risk of heart disease, stroke, cancer and diabetes, lower cholesterol and improve weight management.

This is different from *whole wheat* which typically has been refined. Even though some bran has been added back, this type of grain has lost some of the nutrients in the process. Even so, whole wheat is still a better option than highly processed white breads.

## Protein

*4 Calories per Gram*
*10-15% of Your Daily Calories*

Protein is the basic building block of all life. It helps maintain the body's normal growth process, muscle mass, heart and respiratory functioning and immune system. Each gram of protein you eat provides your body with four calories.

As a general rule, about ten to fifteen percent of the calories you eat in the day should come from protein. If you eat around 2,000 calories per day that is about 200 to 300 calories – around 50 to 70 grams of protein.

How much protein do *you* need? Balancing your protein intake depends on a few factors. If you are pregnant, exercising consistently, recovering from an illness, etc. you need more protein. There is a formula you can use to determine how you are doing with your daily protein intake:

1. Weight in pounds divided by 2.2 = weight in kg
2. Weight in kg x *0.8-1.8* = grams of protein

Notice the range of 0.8 to 1.8 in step two. Use 0.8 in your calculation if you are inactive or a higher number if you are an intense exerciser. Most of us lifestyle-changers fall somewhere in the middle. So, the formula for a 175 pound individual who is exercising a few days a week with a couple days of moderate strength training would look like this:

1. 175 lbs / 2.2 = 79 kg
2. 79 x 1.2 = 94 grams of protein

There is a difference between animal and plant proteins. Meat, poultry, fish, eggs and dairy products are called "complete," meaning they provide all the components for the body to use it most efficiently. Remember to choose leaner cuts of meat and reduced fat dairy foods to reduce your intake of saturated fat.

Plant proteins from seeds, nuts, beans, soy, cereals and grains are incomplete, so they must be combined with another food in order to make a complete protein source. For example, combining beans and rice or bread and peanut butter creates a complete protein.

The following are examples of protein content in various foods:

- One small steak – 52 grams
- One medium chicken breast – 41 grams
- Half can of tuna – 13 grams
- One beef burger – 8 grams
- One cup of milk – 8 grams
- One cheese serving – 7 grams
- Two tablespoons of peanut butter – 7 grams
- One medium egg – 6 grams
- One slice of whole wheat bread – 3 grams

As you can see, the protein content varies greatly in the various foods we eat. The typical American diet provides *plenty* of protein. Remember to choose lean and reduced fat proteins. For example, whole milk and 1% milk provide the same amount of protein, but whole milk has much more fat.

## Fats

*9 Calories per Gram*
*No More than 30% of Your Daily Calories*

Fats are an important component in balanced eating. Each gram of fat you eat provides you with nine calories – more than *twice* the energy you get from a gram of carbohydrate or protein.

Foods like fruits and vegetables have little or no fat while other foods, like butter, are primarily fat. Although you need fat, for the reasons I discussed earlier, some fats are better for you than others. Some should be enjoyed only on rare occasions.

The typical, unbalanced American diet often chooses the wrong types of fats, the kinds that clog the arteries and pack on the pounds. Take the time to educate yourself about the difference in fats and choose to include the healthier sources daily.

- Unsaturated
  These sources of fats are beneficial to your body when consumed in balance. They are found in fish, nuts, seeds and vegetable oils. You may notice unsaturated fats listed on your food labels as monounsaturated or polyunsaturated. Both are beneficial. Some of the best sources of unsaturated fats come from olive oil and fish like salmon.

- Saturated
  Saturated fats remain solid at room temperature and can be found in meats, animal products, cheeses, butter and milk. Eating too much will increase your risk of heart disease. This is why it is so important to reduce your intake of red meat, high fat dairy products and watch the serving sizes of toppings like mayonnaise and butter. Coconut and palm oils, which also contain saturated fats, are used in many baked goods.

- Trans fats
  Fried foods, baked goods, many hot drink mixes such as hot chocolate and gourmet instant coffees and snack foods typically contain trans fats which will be listed as hydrogenated and/or partially hydrogenated fats on the nutrition label ingredients list. One of the most common places to find trans fats is in fast food. Practice moderation when you eat at a fast food restaurant. Trans fats can raise your bad cholesterol levels and decrease your good cholesterol which contributes to heart disease and stroke. Make the

healthy choice to greatly reduce your consumption of trans fats.

The American Heart Association advises that you limit fat intake to no more than thirty percent of your total calories per day. Remember that less than seven percent of your calories should come from saturated fats.

Under these guidelines someone eating around 2,000 calories per day may eat as much as 60 total grams of fat and 15 grams of saturated fat. I encourage the individuals and groups I work with to eat less than the recommended guideline. Read the nutrition label on foods you purchase and ask for a nutrition brochure at your local restaurant to see how your favorite foods stack up.

# Water

The human body is about sixty to seventy percent water. Water is essential for the body to function properly.

Remember the good ol' days when we all drank water right out of the kitchen sink tap? Water used to be the main beverage for most of us when we wanted something to drink. We need to get back to drinking more water and focus on staying properly hydrated.

Don't get tricked into choosing bottled water with added vitamins. Although this is a clever marketing campaign, these popular beverages are not any better for you because they also have added sweeteners and artificial colors.

The better choice is actual water. Choose a water filtration system for your kitchen faucet or a pitcher filtration system sitting prominently on the counter to remind you to drink more water. Six to eight *cups* per day is a good place to start, but you may require more depending on your daily activities and the intensity of your exercise routine.

## Balanced, Achievable Daily Nutrition Goals

There are a few fairly simple nutrition goals I keep in mind every day for myself and my kids. And although I don't always achieve them, I strive for them daily because I know they will benefit us immensely.

- Do not skip meals and eat regularly
  Skipping meals in order to lose weight is still one of the biggest misconceptions around. When you skip meals it sets the stage for impulse buys or a binge before bedtime you will most likely regret later. Eat regularly – graze through your day.

- Balance your meals
  Include carbohydrates, proteins and a little fat in each of your meals. For example, instead of having just cereal for breakfast, add an egg. Eating more balanced meals will assist in regulating your blood sugar and help you feel fuller longer.

- **5** Servings of fruits and vegetables a day
  This is not difficult to achieve when you have your home stocked with healthy items. I strive for 2 servings of whole fruit and 3 servings of vegetables each day. Most individuals I have worked with find this goal realistic and achievable. Personally, I have an apple every day for a snack, a fruit with my lunch and a BIG salad almost every night chock-full of bite-size carrots and broccoli. Your body would benefit even more from whole fruit and vegetables with all the great fiber rather than a fruit juice or high-sodium vegetable drink.

- **6-8** cups of good water per day
  Many of us walk around dehydrated. Your body *needs* water to function properly. Every cell requires it to transport nutrients. Other beverages are fine in

moderation, but strive to drink at least 6 cups of healthy water per day.

## Add More Fiber

One of the best things you can do for your body is to eat foods that are high in fiber. No, not fiber supplements or powders; actual foods that are high in fiber. Eating fiber keeps things moving through your digestive system and may reduce your risk of diabetes and heart disease. Remember to drink adequate water to help this process along. Check your food labels to see how much fiber some of your favorite food items provide. Foods highest in fiber include fruits, vegetables, whole grain breads, cereals and pastas, nuts and seeds.

<u>American Heart Association Guidelines:</u>

Women – 21 to 25 grams per day
Men – 30 to 38 grams per day

## Real Food

We need to get back to eating more real food and less highly processed, individually wrapped items with too many ingredients. If you can't grow your own garden, seek out your local farmer's market. There you will often find organically grown local fruits and vegetables.

Purchasing from local farmers also supports their families and the local economy. Take my advice and visit your local market. Bring your kids and teach them the health and social benefits of buying local. I promise it will become a mainstay for your food selections and a healthy addition to your lifestyle.

## Get off the Blood Sugar Roller Coaster

When you choose to eat in a more balanced way you will begin to feel the benefits immediately.

Balanced eating includes actual eating – yes, eating. Allow me to say again that skipping meals and not eating when you need food is not a healthy and balanced way to lose weight. This method always backfires. You will inevitably end up eating much more later when you have allowed yourself to become ravenous.

Eating five or six small meals a day is much better for your blood sugar and your weight than only eating two or three large meals. People who eat smaller portions typically end up taking in fewer calories overall, experience fewer blood sugar highs and lows and feel much better.

Are you ready to get rid of your highs and lows? Begin by honestly examining the amount of added sugar and highly processed products you are eating and drinking.

*Write it down* if you feel it would help, then make a conscious choice to begin to wean yourself from these foods and beverages. Eating that handful of candy when you are hungry may make you feel satisfied, but it also releases a large amount of insulin into your bloodstream. Riding the blood sugar roller coaster not only affects your mood, but can also cause damage to your body. Choose foods and drinks that create balance, not highs and lows.

## To Sum Up

As you begin to give your body the best fuel it can utilize you will experience the benefits almost immediately. Strive to eat a balance of carbohydrates, proteins and fats at each meal and a variety of real foods throughout your day.

# Chapter 17

# Calories...
# To Count or Not to Count?

*"Never eat more than you can lift."*
*~ Miss Piggy*

The debate over counting calories will continue until the end of time. Both sides of the aisle offer valid points.

One side passionately cites decades of evidence that the calorie-counting movement has made no change in rising obesity numbers in our nation. The other side of the aisle vigorously maintains that we can only gain awareness of what we are consuming by counting our daily food and drink calories.

My view – instead of taking sides, I encourage you to decide for yourself.

I have worked with enough individuals and groups to know that counting calories does not work for everyone. And yet I have known clients who thrive on writing everything down. They may carry a calorie calculator, a handy fast-food slidey guide and a pocket-size journal to record every minute detail of their food and beverage choices.

Then there are those who, for one reason or another choose not to devote any time to counting a single calorie and may focus solely on reducing their portions. I have seen this work well for some people too.

My personal recommendation is that you give it a try, even if just for five days. Grab some measuring cups and spoons and take a few measurements of some of your common foods and drinks to get a realistic picture of what healthier portions look like. Counting your calories should serve to educate you about what needs modification in your daily food and drink choices.

## What is a Calorie?

So, what is a calorie and why do we talk about them so much for weight management?

A calorie is the amount of energy used to raise the temperature of 1 gram of water 1 degree Celsius. And now that I have bored you with the science of it, remember the key word from that definition – ENERGY. Just as in the example of a car running on gas, the foods and drinks we consume provide calories, or energy.

To lose weight, then, eat and drink fewer calories than you are using. Now that you know what calories are, let's discuss why we often blame them for making us fat.

## Empty Calories

Thoughtfully consider your choices when it comes to what you choose to eat and drink. The balanced, real-life approach to reducing your weight and maintaining it focuses on eating less overall, more of what is good for you and exercising regularly.

With that in mind, carefully consider the foods and drinks you eat and drink which serve no other purpose for your body than to provide, what we call *empty calories*. Empty calories typically supply a lot of energy, but provide little or no nutritional value.

A prime example is soft drinks. I like to refer to them as liquid desserts. There is absolutely no nutritive value in cola or sodas, yet the average American consumes hundreds of sodas per year, often in place of the water they should be drinking.

Let's review the typical ingredients: carbonated water, high fructose corn syrup, preservatives, caffeine and artificial colors. One serving provides around 150 to 200 empty calories. Am I saying you should never have another soda? No. If you are going to have an occasional soft drink, make the choice honestly and realize it is an extra – a liquid dessert.

# Change the Way You Look at Calories

How many of us like to talk about calories? I wish everyone could see from my vantage point the reaction on a dozen faces when I introduce a small group discussion about calories. Eyes roll, people move restlessly in their seats, the mood changes. And when I dare to bring up *counting* calories I strategically position myself in front of the nearest exit.

People resist talking about calories because of our old diet baggage. But it's not as bad as you think. Be aware of your self-talk and prepare to change your thinking about calories so you can use this information as a valuable, educational tool.

First, take responsibility for your own actions. Calories cannot make you overweight unless *you choose* to eat and drink too many of them. If you take in more than your body uses it will store the excess as fat. This is exactly why most of us gain around five pounds during the winter months. On top of all the holiday calories we are typically less active, burning off far fewer calories than we are taking in.

When you consume the same amount of calories that you use, your weight will remain relatively stable. Remember that everyone is different, so the number of calories required to lose weight depends on your genetics, how much lean muscle tissue you have, how much you exercise and how active you are through your day.

With that in mind, now is the time to develop an individualized balanced plan to help you on your journey. You will be better able to determine how many calories your body needs in order to begin a balanced half to two pound weight loss per week.

These steps will walk you through a process of self-discovery:

1. Don't change a thing
   I know this may seem odd, but it is very important to begin by taking an honest look at what you are consuming on a regular basis *right now*. For those who want to solidly commit to taking a closer look – *Record* everything, and I mean everything, you eat

and drink for five to seven days. Be sure to include a full weekend in your journal. Read the labels of the things you normally eat, serve yourself what would be a typical portion right now then measure it and record the amount. I know, I know, this will take some time and effort, but it will pay off later. If you want to take it one step further, record the time and any feelings surrounding your choices.

2. Study what you have recorded
   Take an honest look at the patterns and habits that have likely been a part of your lifestyle for years. Do you eat breakfast regularly? How much creamer are you actually putting in your coffee? Is the orange juice you have four ounces, half of a cup, sixteen ounces, two cups? Does the word "fried" appear regularly in your notes? Are the snacks you eat while watching TV every night making up a good part of your days caloric intake? These are the types of questions you want to ask yourself.

   When your goal is a realistic, balanced lifestyle approach to weight management you understand that you don't need to deprive yourself of certain items. But you must begin to honestly examine your habits and accept that some of these may have to change.

3. Add it up
   How many calories, on average, are you realistically taking in per day right now? Most of us underestimate our calorie intake by at least 10 percent, especially on the weekends. Considering your current choices, have you maintained your weight over the past many months, or is your weight increasing? Factor this in as you determine a balanced amount of calories to experiment with as you begin a gradual reduction in your weight.

4. Identify the empty calories

   Pinpoint how many empty calories you are eating and drinking. A healthy lifestyle greatly limits these types of calories. When you do choose these, record them with the letters *EC* to remind you of your choice. Eliminate empty calories first, especially from your home. Are you hitting the vending machine at work regularly? Are you having a second glass of wine with dinner? Limiting or removing these items may be enough to jumpstart your weight loss.

5. Add in the nutrients you are lacking

   Instead of a complete overhaul of your entire eating plan, begin by adding in more fruits and vegetables, good water, whole grains and more fiber. Stock your home with healthier selections and get in the habit of reaching for them when you want a snack.

6. Stop eating a few hours before bed

   This has been debated within weight loss circles for a long time. Why shouldn't you eat before bed? On one hand, it is *not* true that what you eat before bed turns to fat. Remember that weight loss happens when you expend more energy than you take in, so eating at night is not the problem.

   The problem with most of our evening eating is what we're eating and how much. Let's be honest: Most of our evening and midnight snacking does not include fruits and vegetables. No, we typically reach for processed snack foods to eat while watching TV or help us deal with an emotional issue. Not until recently did I commit to cutting out night time eating. I give this lifestyle change partial credit for nudging me off of my recent weight plateau.

You will need to do a little bit of experimenting to discover the best and balanced way for you to eat a little less.

Start by *writing everything down* and striving for around 1500 to 1800 calories per day. You must eat through your day to fuel your body and lose weight in a balanced way. Do *not* drop below 1200 calories per day, especially if you are exercising consistently.

After a few weeks, weigh yourself to see if you are experiencing a balanced half to two pounds per week reduction in your weight. If, after the initial month or so, you are losing more than a couple of pounds a week add some calories back in to your day. Have patience and celebrate even the small reductions.

Remember to focus on the development of healthier lifestyle habits, not dieting. Look at your week as a whole and let go of the urge to be perfect. Eat a variety of foods, watch your portion size and moderate foods and drinks that provide calories, but not nutrition.

If you are not losing weight, even at 1500 calories and exercising, review your food journal and resolve to be completely honest with yourself. Have you been *writing everything down?* If so, and you are still unable to lose weight, talk with your doctor to determine if there are any underlying medical conditions you may not be aware of.

Here are two examples of how an average, balanced intake of calories may look in your day:

1800 Calories per Day
8 servings of bread/starch
6 oz. lean meat/protein
5 servings of fruit
6 or more servings of vegetables
2 servings of dairy (choose lower fat)
3 servings of fat

1500 Calories per Day
6 servings of bread/starch
6 oz. lean meat/protein
4 servings of fruit
5 or more servings of vegetables
2 servings of dairy (choose lower fat)
3 servings of fat

# What is a serving?

As you increase your awareness of the calories you eat and drink, learn to recognize what makes up a serving. Chances are the amounts are a little smaller than you may have imagined. For example, enjoy your pasta at dinner, but be mindful that the 2 cups you dished out on your plate is about 4 servings. Choosing 1 cup may be more balanced as you consider how many servings will benefit your body from that food group in your day.

The following are generalized calorie counts per serving for each food group. Use this as a tool to help you make purposeful choices through your week. Remember to take a few seconds to glance over the nutrition label of the foods and drinks you purchase and see how they compare.

Bread/Starch
(80 calories per serving, choose whole grains)
1 slice of bread or small tortilla (1 ounce)
1/2 bagel or 1/2 English muffin or 1/2 pita
(1 ounce)
1 ounce of ready-to-eat cereal
1/2 cup of cooked cereal, rice, or pasta

Meat/Protein
(55-100 calories per serving, choose lower fat)
1 ounce of cooked lean meat, poultry or fish
(3 oz. is about the size of a deck of cards)
1/4 cup of cooked beans
1 tablespoon of peanut butter
1/2 ounce of nuts
1/2 ounce of seeds
1 egg

Fruit
(60 calories per serving)
1 medium apple, banana or orange
1 cup of berries
1 cup of cubed melon
1/2 cup of chopped, cooked, or canned fruit (no added
    sugar)
1/2 cup of fruit juice

Vegetable

(25 calories per serving)
1 cup of raw, leafy vegetables
1/2 cup of other vegetables, cooked or chopped raw

Dairy
(90-150 calories per serving, choose lower fat)
1 cup of milk
3/4 cup of plain yogurt
1/4 cup of cottage cheese
1 ounce of cheese

Fats
(5 grams of fat and 45 calories per serving)
1 teaspoon oil
1 teaspoon butter
1 teaspoon mayonnaise or cream cheese
1 tablespoon salad dressing

## Portion Size, Portion Size, Portion Size – Did I Mention *Portion Size*?

Managing your weight for a lifetime means learning to enjoy what you eat and drink in moderation without feeling deprived.

Use the following tips to help control your portions and reduce the amount of calories you are taking in a little every day. A few small changes will truly pay off.

- Use smaller dishes
  This is a pretty easy tip. Studies have shown that the larger the plate, the larger the glass, the larger the bucket of popcorn, the larger the container of fries, the more you eat and drink. As much as everything else in our society has been supersized, so have our plates and glasses. Remember the small plates your grandparents used to use? If you can't find a smaller

set of dishes use a dessert size plate instead of a large dinner plate. This applies to beverages as well. Choose the smaller cup for juices. This change alone makes a big difference in the amount of calories you take in through the day.

- Sit down to eat
  Sounds simple enough, doesn't it? Consider how many of us eat in our cars, standing up, sitting in front of the TV or computer. We seem to eat everywhere except the kitchen table. It is hard to control your portions when you are focused on something else. Make the conscious choice to sit down without distraction to enjoy your meal or snack.

- Pack your lunch
  Even when you choose a restaurant that offers healthier selections, the portions will likely be larger than what you would prepare from your home. And what about the drink you order? Those extra calories add up. I have seen many, many people reduce their weight dramatically by changing just this one aspect of their workday routine.

## To Sum Up

Calories give us energy. If you choose to eat and drink too many, you will gain weight. Take a little time to educate yourself about where your calories are coming from and then evaluate where you can increase healthy calories and decrease empty calories. Understand the importance of providing quality fuel for your body. And remember a balanced goal of ½ to 2 pounds of weight loss per week for permanent change.

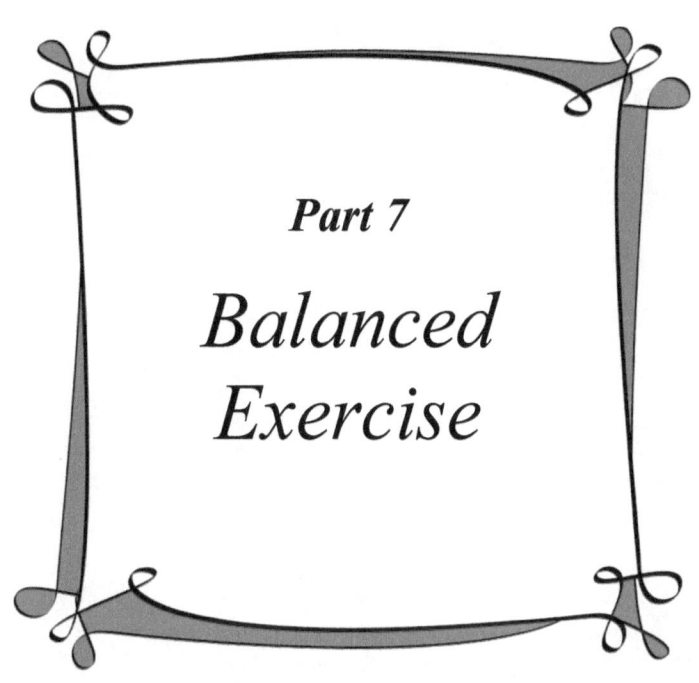

*Part 7*

*Balanced Exercise*

**Chapter 18**

# Exercise...
# The *Key* to Long-Term Weight
# Maintenance

*"Those who think they have not time for bodily exercise
will sooner or later have to find time for illness."*
*~ Edward Stanley*

If you take nothing else from this book, please take this to heart: If you sincerely want to manage your weight and improve your health, make consistent, moderate-intensity exercise a priority.

I cannot stress enough the power this habit will have in changing your life. My goal in this chapter is to make this doable for you. Even if you begin with five to ten minutes of consistent exercise every day you *will* notice a difference.

Use this information to identify one or two exercises you can enjoy as part of your everyday routine. Exercise will steer your journey toward keeping the weight off and will end the cycle of gaining it all, if not more, back.

I have experienced this myself and I have witnessed hundreds of individuals successfully adopt regular exercise after years of ineffective dieting. I have seen how the habit of exercise has drastically changed their lives for the better.

The physical and psychological benefits of exercise are extremely powerful. When you put in the effort to improve your health with exercise, it spreads to other areas of your life – something simply begins to click.

## Benefits of Exercise

Here are just a few of the specific benefits of exercise:

- Exercise burns stored body fat and helps maintain a healthy weight.

- Exercise increases your ability to handle life's stresses.
  The first thing I recommend for stress management is daily exercise. Regular exercise reduces the stress hormones in your body which in turn can lower your blood pressure and your heart rate.

- Exercise improves your mood.
  Consistent exercise actually reduces your chances for depression – dramatically. Instead of reaching for that doughnut when you feel depressed, call a friend to get out and take a walk or jump on your piece of exercise equipment for a few minutes.

- Exercise helps you sleep better.
  Improved sleep is one of the most drastic and immediate improvements individuals experience after adopting the habit of daily exercise.

- Making exercise a priority puts a focus on your health. When you put the time and energy into even a small amount of daily, consistent exercise you feel better about yourself. Use that focus to assist you in making smarter food and drink choices too.

Remember that you are striving for balance. I typically exercise Monday through Saturday and take Sunday off, but there are other times when this schedule is not possible due to circumstances that are beyond my control. Planning to take a day in the week to rest is balanced and can be beneficial so you do not develop injuries from overdoing it. Some people benefit from taking a few days off in a row in the middle of the month. Most of us can admit to taking some time off from our normal exercise routine during a holiday trip or vacation, and that is balanced too.

The benefits of exercise spill into every area of your life, from improved mood to seeing the physical transformation that takes place, exercising consistently encourages you to make healthier choices. Invest the time to develop this life-changing habit.

## Increase Your Activity AND Exercise

"Increase your activity level," is a common phrase among those trying to encourage more exercise and for good reason. Our technologically based society provides increasing energy-saving devices to accommodate every aspect of our lives. We hardly need to move anymore! We drive our car to the corner store, use remote controls for our TVs and spend untold hours in front of our computers. We are simply sitting and less active than *ever before*.

It is no coincidence that our nation's obesity rates continue to increase in direct correlation to the number of channels on our cable TVs. Even small increases in activity can make a difference. Take the stairs instead of the elevator, park further away in the parking lot, walk your grocery cart back into the store after putting your groceries in your car, mow the lawn, walk to school or work. These and many more are excellent ways to increase your daily activity.

Take a moment to write down three small goals that will add a little more activity in your daily life:

1. _____
2. _____
3. _____

## Exercise Cannot Stand Alone For Weight Loss

Remember the general rule of weight loss: unless you have an underlying physical condition, when you eat and drink fewer calories than you use during your day, you will lose weight gradually.

There are many people who try without success to lose weight by dieting and calorie reducing alone. The same is the case for those who try to achieve significant weight loss with exercise alone. Although these individuals begin seeing benefits of exercise such as feeling better, they are sadly disappointed when their efforts do not result in a large reduction in their weight.

Women relate to this much more than men. Men, because they typically have a higher percentage of lean body mass (muscle), often see moderate, immediate weight loss once they start an exercise routine.

For both men and women, though, large and permanent weight reduction rewards will come only once they combine regular exercise with reducing total calories. Both of the pieces must fit together in order to achieve lasting results.

## Three Integral Components of Exercise

My hope is that you will strive to create a balanced exercise routine that will become a positive habit and a daily priority.

Whether you choose to exercise at a local fitness facility, at home or with a buddy, each of the following components of exercise is important. If you are not a member of a fitness facility with trained professionals to assist you, there are many exercise DVDs, cable TV programs, books and websites available to help you develop your individualized routine. These resources should also provide guidance in proper form, safety considerations and illustrations for each aspect.

## 1. Cardio

Cardiovascular exercise; cardio-respiratory exercise; aerobic exercise. All these terms describe exercise that gets your heart pumping, your lungs expanding and your body sweating.

Walking, jogging, swimming, biking, an aerobics class, jump roping – there are dozens of choices when it comes to a good cardio exercise. Exercise is a planned activity. Go ahead and plan some aerobic work into almost every day, just as you would schedule a meal. This approach works.

The American Heart Association (AHA) and the American College of Sports Medicine (ACSM) recommend that adults get 30 minutes of moderate intensity, cardiovascular exercise about five days a week to improve overall health and reduce various disease risks.

If you are someone who chooses vigorous exercise, three days a week for about 20 minutes will provide the same benefit. Kids should be getting about 60 minutes of exercise each day.

Those of us who are trying to reduce our weight, and those maintaining their successful weight loss, 60 minutes most days is almost a necessity. I know that sounds like a lot of planned exercise time each day, but losing weight and subsequently keeping the extra pounds from returning requires extra effort.

The more consistent you are, the easier it is to keep your commitment to exercise. With this said, I will tell you it is balanced to choose one day of the week when you will not work out. And when serious life circumstances arise, and they will, go ahead and take the days or weeks off you need to deal with the crisis. Just strive to get back on track once things have settled down and give yourself time to gradually build up again.

Be careful with this, though. Don't drop your routine lightly. The longer you take a break from your habit the more difficult it can be to get back in the routine. It only takes 48 hours to decrease your ability to handle the exercise level you worked so hard to build up to. Do all you can to make exercise a daily habit.

Always begin each cardio session with a brief warm-up, like walking for a few minutes, followed by a cool-down at the end.

## 2. Strength/Resistance

This aspect of exercise is one many shy away from because they have no idea how to go about it. They may feel it can only be done in a fitness facility setting. Thankfully it is easier than you may think to work strength training into your routine.

Strengthening exercises are very important, especially as we grow older. Unless we do something to maintain our muscle mass, it will decrease as we age, around 1% a year after puberty.

There are many other reasons why you should include this important aspect of exercise:

- Your body uses more energy to maintain and build muscle than fat. Remember the discussion on metabolism – the more muscle you have the higher your metabolism and the more calories you burn, even when you sleep.

- When you strengthen and build muscle you are also increasing bone density, improving your balance, reducing your risk of falls and fractures and toning your muscles for a nicer appearance.

- Strengthening exercises, like all exercise, will reduce your risk for disease and help to manage some diseases as well. Many people with arthritis are surprised by how quickly resistance exercises begin to reduce their pain. Diabetics likewise experience improved glucose levels.

Resistance exercises do not need to be done in a gym. You can benefit from a few easy exercises at home. You can easily do wall or floor pushups, sit-ups and squats using just your body weight as resistance. Also, consider buying inexpensive hand weights and resistance bands from a big-box retailer, local exercise equipment store or online.

Although you can perform cardio exercise every day, strength training needs a different routine.

Work the large muscle groups of your lower body, arms, chest, back and abdomen two times a week. Why not every day? Because your muscles need adequate time to rest and repair between workouts, which means wait about 48 hours before working that specific area again.

Those of us in the fitness field used to exclude the "abs" from this recommendation, but we now understand that the abdominal muscles need recovery time like any other muscle group.

As with aerobic exercise, you should begin and end each strengthening session with a brief warm up and end with a cool down.

## 3. Stretching

Stretching your muscles is an important aspect of exercise. You will benefit from improved flexibility, increased blood flow to the muscles and you may reduce your risk of injury. But stretching is something that should be done properly. Remember these important tips when stretching:

- Do not stretch cold muscles
  It pains me to see someone walk into a fitness facility, sling their leg up onto some piece of equipment, grab their foot and begin stretching. Stretching your muscles before a warm-up can cause muscle injury or strains. I recommend stretching after a warm-up then again at the end of your exercise routine when your muscles are warm.

- Do not bounce
  This technique used to be quite popular. Some of you who have been around the block a time or two may recall this approach to stretching. Turns out, bouncing can cause small tears which may lead to the development of scar tissue within the muscle, making it less flexible.

- Hold the stretch
  Beneficial stretching includes giving the muscle time to actually stretch. Hold each stretch for about 30 seconds and then repeat it again.

- "No pain, No gain" is out
  This old adage should *not* be a part of your exercise routine, especially when it comes to stretching. When you stretch you should feel tension, not pain.

- Be consistent
  Just like cardio and strength exercises, your body will adapt and improve the more consistently you do it. You will experience more and more flexibility the more often you stretch, but will also lose flexibility when you stop.

## Exercise Intensity – The Talk Test

One of the most common questions people ask me as I help them develop their cardiovascular exercise routine is, "How hard should I be exercising?"

I believe the best and simplest way to gauge how hard you are exercising is with the *Talk Test*.

- Light Exercise = You are able to carry on a normal conversation and could even sing a song.

- Moderate Exercise = You are able to talk, but it takes effort. You cannot sing a song.

- Intense Exercise = You have difficulty talking.

After you have built up your ability to exercise continuously for about 10 minutes or more, push yourself to remain in the moderate intensity range for the majority of your cardio routine – you are able to talk, but cannot sing a song. The majority of people will be breaking a sweat when exerting themselves at this intensity. There are no clear benefits to exercising beyond moderate intensity for weight management or overall health benefits.

There are other ways to determine how hard you are working as well. A popular chart you may have seen at your local gym, or if you've ever had a treadmill test, is called the Rate of Perceived

Exertion (RPE) Scale. Some RPE scales run from 1 (no exertion) to 10 (maximal exertion). Others begin at 6 and go up to 20. These are very helpful when documenting results of specific tests, but for the average individual, the Talk Test works very well.

If you are new to exercise you may feel disappointed to hear yourself huffing and puffing as soon as you step on the treadmill or when you go outside for a walk. The good news is that you will improve your endurance quickly if you stick with it. A balanced exercise routine begins slowly. Also, discuss any limitations you have with your doctor and seek guidance from an exercise specialist before starting any exercise program. With time and consistency you will be pleased at your ability to handle a little more each day.

## Your Heart Rate Range (HRR)

As you exercise your heart rate goes up. Although the Talk Test is a helpful and individualized indicator of how intensely you are working during cardiovascular exercise, many people want to know what their heart rate should be while exercising.

For overall health and weight management, "moderate intensity" translates to about 60-70% of your maximum heart rate. To determine your exercise heart rate range use the following formula.

Women: $(226) - (age) \times (60\text{-}70\%)$
Men: $(220) - (age) \times (60\text{-}70\%)$

For example: According to this formula, a 35 year old woman's maximum heart rate range is 191.

$$226 - 35 = 191$$
$$191 \times .6 \sim 115$$
$$191 \times .7 \sim 135$$

Her exercise heart rate range would therefore be about 115 to 135 beats per minute.

As you can see, this formula uses only your age and no other factors so it is not very individualized. It also does not take into consideration any medications you may be on to decrease your blood pressure or heart rate.

Determine how you will take your pulse. This may be easy if you belong to a fitness facility with the latest exercise equipment. Many cardiovascular machines are now equipped with sensors that take your pulse and provide a read-out on the machine.

You can also purchase a chest-strap heart rate monitor at your local exercise equipment store or online. It is accompanied by a wrist device that displays your heart rate.

If neither one of those options are available you can always check your pulse manually by applying your first two fingers gently on the underside of your wrist along the bone on the thumb side. Count the beats for 30 seconds then double that number to determine how many times your heart is beating per minute.

## To Sum Up

As technology and sedentary computer jobs continue to increase we must likewise look for small ways to increase our daily activities every day. Consistent exercise, plus increasing our activity level, is essential to weight management.

Creating a habit of exercise will change your life – I promise you. Over the years I have heard countless people say, "I wish I would have started exercising years ago. Why did I wait so long?" The good news? It is *never* too late to start a daily exercise habit.

**Chapter 19**

# Do *Something* for Exercise

*"You can't make footprints in the sands of time*
*if you're sitting on your butt.*
*And who wants to make buttprints in the sands of time?"*
*~ Bob Moawad, Author*

Time for another dose of truth: I am not going to promise you will fall madly in love with exercise. Some people cannot wait to exercise every day while others learn to tolerate it, but maybe not to the point of *truly* enjoying it.

But there is another truth that's just as important, no matter what group you find yourself in: As you start experiencing the benefits of consistent exercise, you will start asking why you put it off for so long.

Still, despite knowing exercise is good for you; knowing you feel great afterwards; knowing you should be doing it, it can seem so hard to get motivated to exercise! The best piece of advice I can give you is to JUST DO IT. Do *something*!

It is *so* important for you to exercise in order to enjoy good quality of life and maintain your weight that I have devoted this entire chapter to helping you remove your excuses and barriers.

Make exercise a priority and you will reap amazing rewards. Allow the following sections to help you add detail to your goals as you make the commitment to adopt this life-changing habit.

## Start Small

*No* exercise goal is too small. I have encouraged some of my extremely overweight clients to begin with an exercise goal of rolling back and forth in the bed 3 to 5 times. Others I have encouraged to stand beside their bed then sit down on the bed, stand back up, etc. Even walking in place during the commercials of your favorite TV program is accomplishing something. Everyone has to start somewhere, right?

Where are *you* going to start?

Realistically consider what you are physically capable of doing right now, today. If you have never jogged a day in your life, now is not the time to run down to your local recreation center to sign up for next week's 5K run. You are only setting yourself up for disappointment and the likelihood of some expensive medical bills.

A simple walk is a fantastic starting place. If you don't have an area around your home, try visiting a neighborhood park or find a walking trail around your community. Many malls open their doors before business hours to allow the general public to walk laps. My Mom often took advantage of this offering from our local mall. It is an ideal option on hot, rainy or snowy days.

Walking on its own may not burn enough total calories to produce significant weight loss, but it is still a fantastic exercise. As with any other aerobic activity, you will be pleasantly surprised to see how you can push yourself to walk a little bit further each week.

Whether you are new to exercise or adding a new activity in order to mix up your routine, remember to start slowly and then push yourself each day to do a little more. Don't forget to *write down* what you have achieved as it will serve to motivate you and keep you on track.

## No Excuses

As you read through the following common excuses listen carefully to your self-talk. Do not allow excuses to hold you back from developing this life-changing habit. Your new journey will be filled with making realistic, balanced choices. Start by ridding your self-talk of these excuses.

- Exercise is hard – I don't like it.
  Exercise is integral to a healthy lifestyle. If you are serious about improving your health, losing weight and maintaining weight loss, exercise will be a part of your everyday schedule. Finding a balanced routine that works for you personally is your only option, not whether or not to exercise. Remember to start slowly and set small goals that you can achieve right away.

- I'm too busy.
  This excuse simply doesn't hold water. If your health is important to you, you will make the time. How about starting with (3) ten minute small workouts in your day? If you cannot find ten minutes in your day then you need to reevaluate your priorities. Make the time.

- I won't enjoy working out at a gym.
  How do you know if you've never tried it? If you do decide to give it a try, it may be beneficial to choose a facility that will give you a trial period before you sign your name on a contract and commit to a monthly bank draft from your checking account. Even a one-day trial may give you enough of a sample to see if it will fit into your daily routine.

- I don't live near a fitness center and even if I did I can't afford the membership fees so I can't exercise.
  Okay, maybe you cannot afford a gym membership or don't have the time to travel back and forth to the gym, but don't let that become an excuse not to exercise. A home-based exercise program may work best for you. Find a few exercise DVD's, a workout on TV, some simple equipment like a bench step,

jump rope and hand weights or invest in a treadmill or other piece of home equipment that you will use.

There are some people – like me – who exercise at home every day. As a single Mom, tight on time and budget, a gym membership is not something that will fit into my lifestyle. Even when I have worked for various fitness facilities I didn't personally exercise there. I have found a combination of videos and a few pieces of basic, affordable equipment that have stood the test of time. And as I've mentioned, I know realistically that if I don't get my exercise in first thing in the morning there is a 99% chance that it is not going to happen.

My Dad keeps an older model treadmill and weight equipment in his laundry room for those winter days when he cannot make it to the local wellness center. A small TV is mounted to the wall to provide a little entertainment while he works out – this also helps the time pass quickly.

- I can't work out at a gym. I'm self-conscious about how I look.
  You're not the only one. Even the average person may feel intimidated jumping on the elliptical trainer next to a 20-something, size 2 in a little designer exercise outfit. Realize that Miss Size 2 is *not the norm*. Take time to notice all the "normal" people working out. They're just as accepting of you as you are of them.

Avoid comparing your situation with anyone else's. Remember, you're on a journey. You don't have to wait until you can get into a particular bathing suit before joining the water aerobics class at your local recreation center. Imagine if everyone waited to look great in a bathing suit before entering the pool. If that were the case, there would be no water fitness classes!

Almost all exercise facilities welcome members of every age, shape, size and fitness level.

So, have you decided to commit to walking every day during your lunch break at work? Have you decided that you can realistically get up a little earlier each morning to work out with your 30 minute aerobics video? Are you ready to research and compare local exercise facilities in your area?

It does not matter what you choose to do as long as you are doing *something*.

## What Time is Right?

Life is busy and no matter how long you wait for it, the Time Fairy is not going to show up with her magic wand and grant you ten, thirty or sixty minutes of free, uninterrupted time to exercise. You have to *make* the time.

Begin by pinpointing the time of day when you have the most energy. One of the BIGGEST mistakes people make when setting an exercise goal is choosing the wrong time of day. If you try to take on a new task when you are exhausted you will end up skipping it until you finally give up entirely.

If you are one who has to drag yourself out of bed in the morning, but you feel your engine revved up by lunchtime, then a membership to your local gym may be a good fit for you.

On the other hand, if you wake up in the morning with energy and motivation, knowing that you will get more tired as the day goes on, a morning home exercise routine may work well for you.

Everyone is different and there is no cookie-cutter solution. Take the time to think about what time of day you will be most likely to exercise.

## Do You Need a Buddy?

It is important to ask for help and support when you need it.

For extra encouragement, seek out a friend or relative for support and a swift kick in the pants when you need it. An exercise buddy is one of the best support systems you can have. Your buddy will be there to say, "Hey, what time are we going for our walk?" or "What time should I swing by and pick you up so we can head to the gym?"

During your shared exercise time you can encourage each other to push it just a few more steps or minutes.

One of the best benefits of a fitness buddy is simply the opportunity to share and talk. This is not only therapeutic, but it helps the time pass faster and makes the experience that much more enjoyable.

## Would You Benefit From the Help of a Personal Trainer?

So, you have joined a fitness center. You have no clue where to begin and need some help setting up an exercise program. Maybe you are ready for some professional guidance as you seek a balanced routine that meets all your needs. A personal trainer can be a valuable addition to your exercise routine. Many facilities offer free services if you pay a monthly fee, so take advantage of the professionals' advice as much as possible.

First, determine what you are looking for in a trainer. Are you going to be more comfortable in a gym setting or at home? Would you prefer a male or female trainer? There are many options available to you, but make sure you do your research carefully before deciding which route to take and who you will hire.

Personal training has developed into a lucrative business over which there is little if any official monitoring or standards, so ask the important questions and choose wisely.

In order to make the most educated choice, use the following tips to help you hire the right person:

- Education and Certifications
  If you are a member of a reputable fitness facility, like a YMCA, you can be assured that the employees in the fitness center hold certifications and receive continuing education to keep their certifications up to date. You may not receive that same guarantee from a

smaller, independent gym or freelance trainer. Do not make the common mistake of equating big muscles with an expertise in fitness training.

- Ask for a referral and observe
Ask around. Word of mouth will be your best referral source. If you are a current member of a fitness facility and have the opportunity, watch how the trainers interact with clients to see if they are attentive and compatible with a variety of personalities.

- Safety
A qualified trainer will hold current certifications in CPR and First Aid. You want to know that the person providing you with that extra nudge in your exercise routine will be prepared in case of an emergency, especially in your home.

- Are they interested in *your* goals?
The first session with your trainer must include both time to discuss your personal goals and a thorough assessment of your current fitness status. If it doesn't, walk away. Do not be afraid to speak up if you feel you are not being heard. I have witnessed far too many "trainers" throw someone on a piece of equipment, set the speed, hit the start button and walk away without carefully considering the person's ability level or fitness goals. Your trainer should understand that everyone is different and that there is no one-size-fits-all exercise prescription.

- What should you pay?
Before you sign a contract with a trainer do your research. Make some phone calls and compare pricing. Trainers who come into your home will typically charge more than those working at the local gym, depending on their credentials. Also, exercise physiologists, who are personal and athletic trainers

with a masters or bachelors degree, will charge more for their services. Such an expert may be a good fit if you are looking for someone to guide you in a specific sport or expand your current routine.

## Get the Right Gear

How important is having the right attire and footwear for your workout? Very important. If you are going to start a walking program, make sure you have a good pair of walking shoes. If you are going to mix up your workout a quality pair of cross trainers will work well. Be prepared to invest some money in the proper footwear for the activity you choose in order to protect yourself from pain and injury.

Breathability is also a necessity. It still amazes me to see someone walk into a gym wearing one of those "plastic" sweat suits from the 1970's. You know the ones I'm referring to. They resemble something from an old sci-fi movie. The zipper is tucked right under the chin and the suit sports thick elastic around the wrists and ankles to encourage maximum sweat. Throw those old suits away! Long gone are the days of encouraging you to sweat buckets in order to lose weight. That kind of weight loss is merely water loss and those pounds return as soon as a person begins drinking fluids again.

Most importantly, be comfortable. There are no fashion police at your local fitness facility. The right shoes and comfortable clothing will make your daily exercise habit that much easier.

## I'm Bored!

Are you tired of hitting your DVD's play button on the same old exercise video? Do you dread stepping on the elliptical trainer one more time?

While some people can keep up their walking routine or trip to the gym without getting bored, a lot of us need to mix it up in order to keep things interesting. Becoming bored with the same old routine is not uncommon, especially if you exercise indoors on equipment.

Try one or two of the following tips to ensure your exercise routine stays interesting:

- Try something completely different
  If you have always exercised on your own at home, consider adding a membership at one of your local community fitness centers. It is difficult to become bored when there are so many activities to choose from, like swimming and group exercise classes and where you can regularly meet new friends. How about joining the local volleyball league or your church's softball team?

- Get outside
  As I have previously mentioned, take advantage of the outdoors. Join a tennis group in your area; find a walking, biking or hiking trail where you can enjoy the therapeutic benefits of being outside.

- Add on to what you are already doing
  It may be time to add more time or another dimension to your exercise routine. Are you currently incorporating daily cardiovascular exercise? Getting in your two or three days of moderate strength training exercises? Stretching after your routine? If you are skipping any of these three components now is the time to add it in.

- Ask the advice of a professional
  A personal trainer will encourage you to incorporate a variety of routines in order to keep you from getting bored with the same old program. Being accountable to a professional will also motivate you to stick with it.

## To Sum Up

Exercise is important to a healthy lifestyle, but an absolute necessity for weight maintenance. Start small and slow to set yourself up for success. Do not allow yourself to make excuses – just do it and you'll be happy you did. Choose something you can and will do consistently and then make it a part of almost every day of your life.

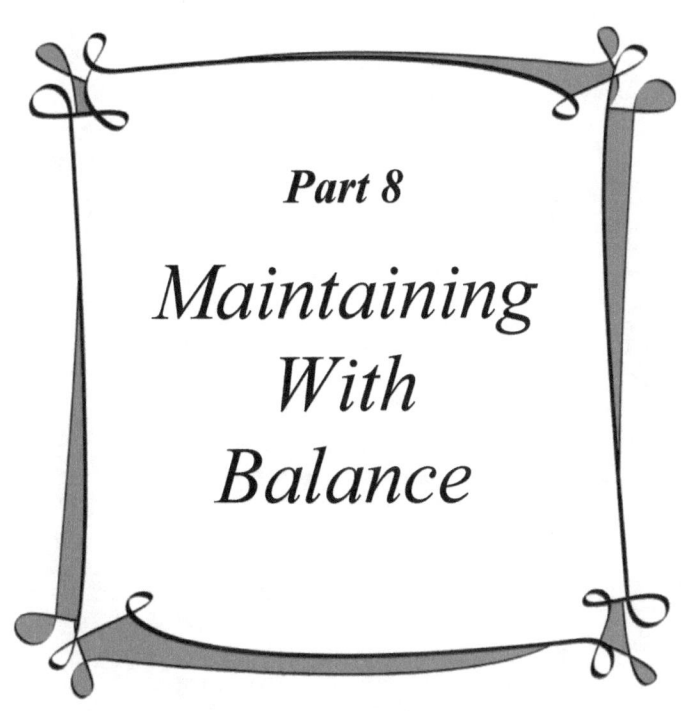

*Part 8*

# *Maintaining With Balance*

# Chapter 20

# No Need to Reinvent the Wheel

*"There are three kinds of men.*
*The one that learns by reading.*
*The few who learn by observation.*
*The rest of them have to pee on the electric fence*
*to see for themselves."*
*~ Will Rogers*

I don't know about you, but I would prefer to be included in one of the first two groups of guys described by Mr. Rogers. Learning from the hard work and mistakes of others is sure a lot easier than having to go through the struggles and mistakes for ourselves.

Allow me to remind you again of the fine print at the bottom of the screen of practically every single weight loss infomercial and supplement advertisement:

*Results not typical.*
*Participants also included a reduced calorie*
*and exercise program.*

The results you see are *not* typical. Most of the weight-loss advertisement models in these ads have never even tried the product. The few actual participants pictured worked to eat smarter, eat less and exercise in order to achieve results.

Advertisers will continue to come along, angling for your money by repackaging weight loss equipment, supplements and programs with bells and whistles to make it sound newer and better, but it is not.

You do not need that supplement with its accompanying side-effects. You do not need to tailor your foods based on your blood-type or body shape. You do not need to purchase that shiny piece of exercise equipment unless you are actually committed to using it for something other than a place to hang your clothes.

What you need to do is realize that the time has come to let go of the quick gimmicks and commit to honest, realistic and manageable changes that, in time, will reap huge rewards for your mind, body and spirit. Having this knowledge should empower you to stop relying on someone or something else to come along and fix you. Learn from those who have done it the right way and succeeded.

## National Weight Control Registry

We know what it takes to reach a healthier weight range. Eating smarter and eating less overall, coupled with a commitment to exercise, works. If you would like more solid evidence, check out the *National Weight Control Registry* at www.nwcr.ws.

The Registry was created to determine how people lose weight, and even more importantly, how they maintain that loss for the long-term. Originally created in 1994 by two doctors, the database now includes over 10,000 individuals who have lost significant amounts of weight and have *kept it off.*

Here are some of the interesting, current findings gathered from the participants:

- 98% report that they modified their food intake in some way to lose weight

- 94% increased their physical activity, walking being the most frequently reported form of activity

- 90% exercise, on average, around one hour per day

- 78% eat breakfast every day

- 75% weigh themselves at least once a week

- 62% watch less than ten hours of television per week

Another interesting finding is that about 55 percent of those registered said they achieved their success with the help of a support group while 45 percent did it on their own.

These statistics come from thousands of individuals who decided it was time to make a change in their lives and take responsibility for their personal choices. Each one of those registered has their own unique story of how they came to the realization and readiness to make real-life, lasting changes in their thinking and choices which will benefit them for a lifetime.

## Modifying Your Food Intake

First, notice that almost 100 percent of those registered report reducing their calories.

Hopefully, by now, you understand that dieting does not work for the long-term. Gradual new habits in your eating will make the biggest difference over time. Remember, you did not gain your excess body weight overnight, so be patient with yourself as you add some healthier foods choices and reduce some not-so-healthy food and beverage selections in most of your days.

Moderation and portion control are vital to the adoption of a balanced lifestyle. There is no need to eliminate completely all the foods you enjoy. Begin by focusing on eating less and adding in what you know will provide your body what it needs to make you feel good.

Putting in the effort to make gradual change will lead to modifying some of your other food and drink choices.

## Keep Recording

Keep yourself accountable by grabbing your journal or notebook when you find yourself veering off track and reaching for your larger jeans. It may seem time-consuming, but it is one of the most valuable maintenance tools you have at your disposal.

If you can identify as an emotional eater, keep your journal handy daily to record why you are eating and recognize that you are in control of your choices. Do not look to food to solve any of the stresses or trials you are going through. You know you will regret it later.

Be honest. Remind yourself that no one is perfect – no one. Begin right where you are and take it one day at a time. Look forward as you give yourself a break and focus on the positives.

## Eat Breakfast

Breaking your fast is important for your body and your mind. Sadly, breakfast is often the easiest meal to skip in the day. Did you know that people who are overweight are more likely to skip breakfast than those who are a healthier weight?

Taking that even further, those who only eat a couple of large meals tend to be heavier than those who eat smaller, more frequent meals throughout the day.

Skipping any meal is not healthy and will not help you lose weight. As a matter of fact, it will make weight loss more difficult since you tend to eat more at your next meal because you are so hungry. Not to mention the impulse junk food snack buys from the convenient vending machine, to help you get to the next meal.

Make breakfast a priority in your day.

## Why Daily Exercise?

94 percent of those surveyed in the Weight Loss Registry report increasing their physical activity and 90 percent continue to make it a priority for an hour a day in order to maintain a healthier weight.

You eat every day, you get dressed every day; you have many daily habits you would never consider skipping. A consistent, daily exercise routine must become just as important as any other daily habit. It is even more important if your goal is to maintain a healthy weight.

60 minutes is a good chunk of time out of each day, but a necessity if you are trying to reduce your weight significantly. I have noticed consistently that the more weight someone has to lose, the more exercise must be a daily and often timely ritual.

In my experience as a Wellness Coach, I cannot recall one client who stopped exercising cold-turkey who did not gain most or all of the weight they lost back, *plus more*. Remember to have balance and remain flexible.

When exercise is an important priority in your life and has become a daily habit, it is much easier to get back on schedule when your routine has been interrupted. Return to your normal routine before too much time passes.

## Keep It Up for All the Right Reasons

If you have not done so yet, take the time to *write down* why you need and want to lose weight. Post it in a location where you will see it every day – maybe on your bathroom mirror or your computer at work.

Remind yourself daily of the reasons why making your health a priority is important to you and to your loved ones.

- Recall often the importance of the connection of your mind, body and spirit.

- Believe that you will succeed.

- Make the time to breathe and pray.

Chapter 21

# Did You Fall Off the Wagon
# or
# Did you Eat the Wagon?

*"It's not whether you get knocked down;
it's whether you get up."*
*~ Vince Lombardi*

If there is one guarantee I can give you about your journey to manage your weight, it is that you will not only slip up along the way, but occasionally experience complete face plants as you strive to fit healthier choices into your lifestyle. That's life.

You will, on occasion, lapse back into some of your old habits or not commit the time to your balanced goals. Life issues will arise that are completely out of your control. The best thing you can do is to prepare yourself for the inevitable lapse.

Coach Lombardi was exactly right – it comes down to your personal decision to get back up or not. Remember, it is your choice. No more excuses.

## The Difference Between Lapsing and Collapsing

Lapses are bound to happen, because life happens. The illness or loss of a loved one, a crisis with your job or one of a million other life trials and changes will occur eventually. We cannot control every aspect of life to accommodate an ideal, healthy lifestyle.

As an example, I recently cared for a dear friend as she came to the end of her life. She was 96 years old and had no family. I found myself spending hours with her at the nursing home every day, while also trying to be present for my job and at home for my two sons. I hardly slept, I ate standing up most of the time and my exercise routine flew out the window.

When my friend passed away many months later, I had no regrets. Yes, I had gained weight, yes, my body felt the effects of not exercising for that time, but I make no excuses for my decision and was blessed by the time we spent together at the end of her life.

After some time had passed I made the choice to get back on track. It took a while to get my routine going again, especially as I grieved, but exercising helped me through that process too.

Life happens. This is why I stress that you should not strive for perfection, because you will constantly feel disappointed in yourself. A balanced, realistic focus will allow you to ride the waves of life as they come and go.

To help you get back on track when you lapse, remember your priorities. Your health and self-care should be one of the top numbers on that list. Committing to small behavior changes and daily exercise makes a full collapse back into an old, unhealthy lifestyle less likely. Once most people experience the benefits of healthier eating and exercise they may lapse occasionally, but rarely fully collapse.

A change in lifestyle with a clear understanding of moderation and balance makes the journey realistic. Unlike an unbalanced approach in which someone goes "on" or "off" of a diet, a lifestyle approach looks at the big picture – focusing on the long-term.

## The Plateau

There are few things more frustrating than when you have worked hard to change your eating and exercise habits only to hit a plateau. Your weight has been dropping consistently but now you suddenly can't get it to budge. You are stuck.

It has happened to all of us. Do not give up when you hit a plateau. Use the following points to help you evaluate what is going on and what changes or additions you can make to get the ball rolling again.

- Give it time
  Keep in mind that balanced weight loss averages around ½ pound to 2 pounds per week. The more weight you have to lose, the more loss you will experience in the beginning. Remind yourself that you did not put on the extra pounds overnight. The slower you take the weight off, the more likely your loss will be permanent, IF you have committed to a daily exercise routine. Waiting is hard, but you will continue to see your investment pay off with an improved quality of life.

- Evaluate your weight loss goals
  When one of my clients says they have hit a plateau I always begin with a discussion of their goals. Specifically, how much weight do they feel they should lose and is this realistic? Is your own goal realistic? If you feel convinced that you should weigh 120 pounds, but have never weighed less than 140 in your adult life, your body may be trying to tell you something. Have you hit a plateau or has your body reached a comfortable and healthy range?

- *Write it down* again and again and again
  This is one of the best tools to assist you in managing your weight. Keep yourself honest and accountable. Pull out your journal or notebook. Invest the time to record what is going on for a few days. Evaluate where empty calories may have gotten back in or where you can reduce or eliminate them. Are you eating breakfast? Are your portions balanced? Are you eating before going to bed? The goal is not to be

as strict as possible, but to see where you can make small changes to keep your energy intake in check.

- Exercise – Change it Up
  If you are not currently exercising and have tried to reduce your weight by modifying your eating, you need to add this important component to your day. Without exercise you will likely gain the weight back, plus more. Now is the time to make it a daily habit. If you are already exercising then it may be time to mix things up a bit. Your body may be used to your current routine. You might benefit from something different. Try investing in a local fitness center membership and add the help of a professional to your program. You can also try breaking up your exercise session into two parts in your day.

- Exercise – Make the Time
  You may be exercising, but is it enough? You may need more time and/or more intensity. Remember that exercise alone is not that effective for many people in reducing their weight significantly, but it is integral to building and maintaining lean muscle tissue and maintaining weight loss. For example, your walking routine may need to increase by adding another day each week, more distance and some more gitty up in your step. Strive to reach a level of moderate intensity where you are still able to talk, but have to work at it. Make sure you are working up a sweat and push yourself a little more each day.

## Lessons from the Past

Growing up in my home it was tradition to sit down for at least two family meals every day – unheard of in most homes today. My Mom, a saint, made a cook-to-order breakfast practically every morning. Every supper included a salad, vegetable, meat, starch and dessert – all served family-style. I can still smell the homemade bread and yeast rolls being pulled from the warm oven. And yes, we were told to finish everything on our plates because there were "starving children in China who would be happy to have it."

We enjoyed many organic products before eating organic was the "in" thing. Most of the locals ate organically when I was growing up; it was commonly referred to as "gardening." Many of us also paid or traded for various foods from neighbors who raised cows and chickens.

Our delicious milk and eggs came from the Edmisten Farm. My Mom and Lola would visit for a while before we loaded one or two glass gallon jugs capped with plastic wrap and a rubber band into the car for transport home. Before we drank the milk Mom would skim off the cream for coffee. Our yard was too sloped and rocky for planting, so we raised our large garden on a borrowed plot at the Edmisten's. As a young girl it often seemed tiresome to cram all seven of us in the car, drive down the road and work in that garden. We would plant seeds, toss out rocks and pull weeds until the sun set over the Blue Ridge Mountains. I remember falling asleep to the sound of Mom sterilizing jars and canning vegetables late into the night. We enjoyed those home grown vegetables for months afterwards. Today I cherish those memories.

As an active kid in the Appalachian mountains of North Carolina it was easy to burn off all those delicious calories. We played outside – that's what everyone's kids did. Especially since our TV only received three channels and one was fuzzy unless we had our youngest brother, Kent, scoot around in his footy pajamas and hold the antenna.

The closest neighbors with children were over a mile away, down the mountain from where we lived, so my siblings and I primarily played together. My older brother, David, built ramps for us to ride our bikes over.

And although there were more than a few times in my childhood when I was called "chubby" (as we used to refer to it back then), my brothers, sister and I stayed so active hiking, skiing, and riding our bikes that we never even gave a second thought to our weight. We had physical education every day in school and practically everyone was involved in the local parks and rec sports teams all year. We would also often walk from the school up the street to our town park and play tag, four-square, tether ball, jump rope, basketball and swing on the swing sets for hours. Most of us walked home from the bus stop. Our hike was more than a mile – literally uphill.

To say that "times have changed" would be one of the greatest understatements of our evolving society. Families no longer eat together and if they do, it is often in front of the TV, not around the family table. Meals are typically purchased from a restaurant instead of prepared at home. Food and drinks are often consumed while standing up or driving in a car to some activity or event. And even though I am rearing my children in the same small town where I grew up, I, like the majority of parents, am too concerned for safety to send them out to play alone in our community park today.

Although our local school provides physical education every day, most schools in our nation do not. PE has either been cut from the curriculum or reduced to a weekly handful of minutes in many of our public schools.

So, knowing that we must move forward on our journey, where can we go from here?

## Go Back for the Future

For our health's sake, and for the health of future generations, we must learn to simplify our lives and find the balance.

We must first understand the power we have given away to those who are only interested in making money off of us. Take control and educate yourself so you can make better decisions for yourself. Do not believe every weight loss claim you see and hear. Most importantly, love and respect yourself enough to accept responsibility for your own health.

We need to sit down and take time to savor most of our meals, whether we are alone or with our family. We need to eat more raw foods, less highly processed foods and drink healthy water instead of soft drinks.

We need to unplug from our electronics. We need to get up and move in many small ways to increase our activity. We need to find time to be still and enjoy the outdoors. Can any of us even comprehend what a day without a TV or computer would be like? Recognize how much time and money we spend entertaining ourselves and turn some of that around as we use our gifts to help others.

Remember the simpler times of the past and integrate some of those positive aspects back into your daily life again. Think about some small changes you can make today, right now, that will make a positive impact on your health, your family's health and help your community.

You have what it takes to refocus your priorities and bring balance into your life. The choice is yours.

# Recommended Resources:

*Nutrition Action Newsletter*
Produced by the *Center for Science in the Public Interest* (CSPI). Offering the latest, unbiased nutrition information for healthy living with no advertisements.
www.cspinet.org/nah

*SparkPeople*
FREE online support community offering recipes, exercise guidance, personal goal tracking and motivation from the privacy of your own home.
www.sparkpeople.com

*Zonya Foco, RD*
Creator of DIET FREE – the most balanced, educational and reality-based nutrition program available today.
www.zonya.com

*National Weight Control Registry*
Over ten thousand have registered and shared what works to maintain their weight loss. Let their success stories encourage you to keep going.
Phone: 1-800-606-NWCR (6927)
www.nwcr.ws

Dr. Ramani Durvasula
Special thanks for sharing your personal journey with all of us.
www.doctor-ramani.com

*Overeaters Anonymous*
*"I put my hand in yours, and together we can do what we could never do alone."*
Ask for help when you need it. Locate this valuable support network in your local area. Members respect each other's anonymity and all meetings are confidential. If you cannot make a face-to-face meeting or are uncomfortable joining a group in person, OA offers meetings online and over the phone.
www.oa.org

Eat Smart, Move More NC
A healthy lifestyle means eating smarter and moving more. North Carolinian's source for sound information.
www.eatsmartmovemorenc.com

# Notes

Chapter 2
1. McMillan, Matt. "Study: Most obese moms, kids underestimate their weight." *Health.com*. Cable News Network, 24 March 2011. Web. Jan. 2012.

Chapter 4
1. Bartlett, Ph. D, Susan. "Role of Bodyweight in Osteoarthritis." *Hopkinsarthritis.org*. The John Hopkins Arthritis Center, 27 March 2012. Web. July 2012.

Chapter 5
1. Othersen Gorman, Megan. "Thinking 'I'm Just Big Boned' Could Be Keeping You Fat." *Rodale.com*. Rodale. Web. January 2012.

Chapter 10
1. Adams, K., Lindell, K., Kohlmeier, M., Zeisel, S. "Status of nutrition education in medical schools." *Am J Clin Nut*, April 2006, Vol. 83, No. 4.

Chapter 11
1. Gallagher et al. *Am J Clin Nut*, 2000; 72:694-701

Helpful Informational Resources:

*National Institutes of Health (NIH)*
Phone: 301-496-4000
www.nih.gov

*Centers for Disease Control and Prevention*
Phone: 800-CDC-INFO
www.cdc.gov

*American Heart Association*
Phone: 800-AHA-USA-1
www.americanheart.org

*Diabetes Research & Wellness Foundation*
Phone: 202-298-9211
www.diabeteswellness.net

*National Heart Lung and Blood Institute*
Phone: 301-592-8573
www.nhlbi.nih.gov

*National Cancer Institute*
Phone: 800-4-CANCER
www.cancer.gov

Special Thanks
Dr. Lila Bauman, Editor
Kerri Ledford, Photographer

www.ingramcontent.com/pod-product-compliance
Lightning Source LLC
Chambersburg PA
CBHW061402280526
45784CB00001B/337